My Essential Oils Just Arrived! Now What?

The 1, 2, 3's and A, B, C's for New Essential Oil Users

Dr. Sandra G. Smith, EdD

My Essential Oils Just Arrived! Now What?

The 1, 2, 3s and A, B, Cs For Beginning Essential Oil Users

Copyright © January 2015 Dr. Sandra G. Smith, EdD

Dr. Sandra Smith at Sandra@drsandragsmith.com

The content of this book is for general instruction only. Each person's physical, emotional, and spiritual condition is unique. The instruction in this book is not intended to replace or interrupt the reader's relationship with a physician or other professional. Please consult your doctor for matters pertaining to your specific health and diet.

To contact the publisher, or the author, email Sandra@drsandragsmith.com

ISBN: 978-0-9963266-0-5 (Print/paperback)

Printed in the United States of America

To all of my friends and family who also love and share essential oils with others! Thanks for teaching me!

CONTENTS

ACKNOWLEDGMENTS

I would like to acknowledge the support and encouragement of the wonderful group of essential oil users and experts from whom I have learned so much and whom I have grown to love since I began my own journey into this exciting world. I'd also like to thank my family for their patience as I have put many other things on the back burner in order to complete this project.

A Short History of Medicine:

"Doctor, I have an earache."

2000 BC: "Here, eat this root."

1000 BC: "That root is heathen. Say this prayer."

1850 AD: "That prayer is superstition. Drink this potion."

1940 AD: "That potion is snake oil. Swallow this pill."

1985 AD: "That pill is ineffective. Take this antibiotic."

2000 AD: "That antibiotic has side effects. Here, take this root."

(~ Author anonymous)

1 INTRODUCTION

You've been checking the porch expectantly waiting for your oils to arrive. You LOVE the orange essential oil that you received at the class you attended where you decided you needed more and so you placed your order. Mmmmm….It smells wonderful! You know that it is like gold – seems magical even – but you don't remember much more. There was so much that they told you about in the class you attended.

Now, you can't wait until your box arrives! It will be wonderful to have helpful natural options for helpful natural options for your family's health and wellness right at your fingertips! You were so impressed by the many ways that essential oils can benefit you and your family; now you can't wait until you have them in YOUR home! Your friend who shared her oils with you said that it would be nice if each home had essential oils on hand for a variety of reasons. All were about helping the body heal itself in some way. That was what struck a chord inside you!

Finally, you check the front porch and the package is there!

How exciting! Your oils have arrived!

You open the box. Wow! So many shiny, new, amber bottles! You notice the label on each oil that tells you a little more about it. You are curious…! And excited…! You notice the name of each one. You have an idea about some uses for some of them. Inside the box, there is a little information about them. You read the information there. There may be some suggested possible uses for each one. It's not a lot of information, but it seems difficult to keep track of each one and how it is different from the next one. As you move from one to the next, you begin to forget what you just read about the previous oils as you focus on the current bottle.

Perhaps you were given a guide of some kind to help you. Perhaps you watched videos about them. Wow! There is so much to remember and keep straight! Each essential oil has the potential to support your family's health in so many ways! It is important and you want to remember, but it's like a different language.

How is it that you seem to know about what to eat or not, or what to do for common health issues or first aid using some basic things in your home, but you can't remember very much about the essential oils, how to use them and which is for what? If you think about it, you realize that you learned about many of these things as they were used on you through your childhood and over your lifetime, so you decide not to be discouraged. Soon, you will become well versed in the essential oils, too, and which ones help you and your family's health needs best. At least you hope you will!

You look at the papers you saved from the class where you ordered the oils. As you look at your new bottles of oils, read about them and then smell them, it seems like you are beginning to remember a few things. You know that when you first smelled the peppermint, you had a reaction – a positive one! You remember the lady in the class who talked about her story.

It could have included anything as each person has his/her own story.

Perhaps she had a number of medical issues and after being told western medicine could only do so much, she felt that the oils helped support her body in its recovery. Perhaps she found a quick solution that was helpful in promoting calming, or soothing and helping her sleep. Perhaps he noticed that he used to get sick every winter and now he doesn't, and attributes that to taking supplements, or when he does, it is not as bad, or it doesn't last as long as it used to. Perhaps you know of teachers who have noticed that diffusing essential oils in their classroom makes it easier for them to manage their students.

But now this is about you and your family! Where do YOU begin? How will the use of essential oils impact YOUR life? How will it help YOUR family and the people that you know or meet?

It's exciting to think about! And it might make you curious, doubtful, or anxious. Or maybe something in between.

What do other people do? You know that they "use" essential oils, but how, when and for what? Do they use them everyday? Do they use them for specific things? How much do they use? Where should you begin?

Maybe you are afraid to open them up! Or maybe you want to save them because, after all, you just spent a lot of money on them. When is the last time that you bought an entire supply cabinet of supplements, health aids, or health care products - all at once?! It was a chunk of money! You value these precious little bottles! You don't want to waste them!

But part of you wants to try them each out! So, you give in. I'm going to use them! Someone told you that they used essential oils everyday. Everyday?! How would you do that?

There are so many questions that are bound to come up that I suggest that you invest in a good book that includes information about many more essential oils and blends than you think you will need. You can find many online or through essential oils retailers.

Having something basic first is a good idea. Often they will give you plenty of research and background about many essential oils and about specific health concerns or issues, body systems and how they can best be supported, soothed or helped. There are also specific books that review the use of essential oils for emotional healing, guidance with chakras, or releasing emotional patterns with the use of essential oils. There are books that discuss where essential oils are mentioned in the Bible. There are many other resources available but these will get you started.

You may, if you are a science geek like me, even want to research PubMed, where hundreds of thousands of research studies are published for your review. Honestly, I didn't think that I would do it, but as I found my essential oils to be so beneficial to myself and my family, I became fascinated by them. I did go back and was excited to learn about the history and origins of known use of essential oils, and about the early scientists and pioneers in the exploration of essential oil use.

The purpose of this guide is to help you get started using *your* essential oils - the oils you selected first - including whether to use them topically, aromatically, or internally, where to put them when you use them topically, how much to use, how often to use them, and other basics about using your brand new set of essential oils!

You will also find guidelines here for essential oils you will want to have on hand to support the various body systems in times of stress or upset and when you would use them. However, for your own specific health issues or concerns, you will want to do a bit of research in order to find the perfect auxiliary essential oils and supplements for your health and wellness.

As experts on essential oils say, when you begin using and learning about essential oils, many have life changing results. I hope that this will be your experience!

I imagine you still have many questions. Are essential oils safe? Are they effective – do they work? What should you expect? When you shared with others that you spent money on some essential oils, did you get questions or raised eyebrows? Did you begin to second-guess your decision?

Let me ease your mind. If anyone around you gives you a "thumbs down" or wants proof as to the efficacy of essential oils, all they have to do is go to PubMed, the U. S. National Library of Medicine's database, and do a search. There have now been tens of thousands of studies done that support the natural healing properties of the essential oils.

Many of us want to integrate natural or alternative medicine options with what our current healthcare options. Modern medicine relies on technology and pharmacology, which can be life saving, but can also have disastrous health implications. Sometimes we just have to take the bad (side effects) for the good benefits.

In the realm of natural health solutions, essential oils reign supreme for a variety of reasons including:

- Benefits to body, mind / emotion, and spirit
- Most have an indefinite shelf life

- Versatility and adaptability – one oil can be used for many purposes adapting to a body system as needed
- Extremely potent compared to herbs from the same plant source
- Safe – with minimal contraindications when used sparingly
- Easy to use – dosing and application have wide margins for error.

In our family, we have been using essential oils for the past few years and have benefitted from them in the following ways:

- They have provided us with digestive support
- They have provided us with seasonal support when pollens and other allergens are abundant
- They have helped us by improving lung function
- They have helped us have improved sleep
- Our immune systems have been boosted
- Our skin is healthier
- We have more energy
- We have been able to repel insects and support our bodies in treating insect bites and stings
- Our pets have benefitted from them in a variety of ways!

As you can see, we have gained a great deal by adding essential oils to our regimen for healthcare. I hope that our experiences and those of our friends will give you some ideas into how you can also benefit by using essential oils in your families!

2 WHERE TO BEGIN: THE 1, 2, 3'S OF USING ESSENTIAL OILS

Let's begin at the beginning! You have your oils, now...

1) Open up the Bottles

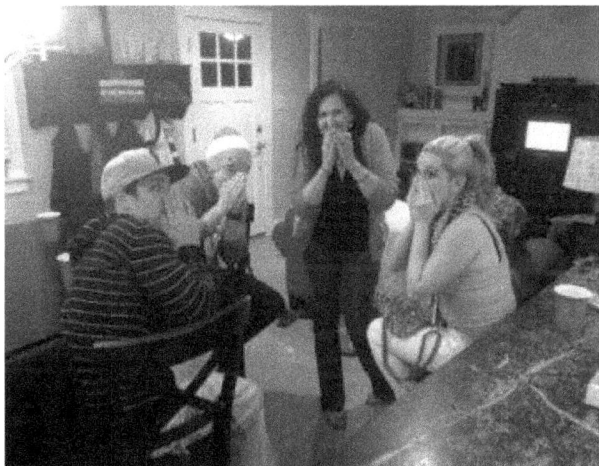

Smell your oils! Open your bottles one by one and smell each of these precious oils, each one of which is such a gift! My favorite method for smelling my essential oils is to put a drop in my hand, rub hands together, and cup hands over my nose and breathe in.

Close your eyes and just be in the moment, experiencing the effects of each unique scent. Think of its name and the plant that provided its essence for your use. I like to look at a picture of the plant to help me in this imagining moment.

Share the experience with someone you care about! The picture above is of me with a couple of my grandchildren. I was sharing orange, one of my favorites, with them! They loved the experience, too!

Take your time. Pay attention to the oils that appeal to you most. Notice the ones that appeal to you the least. Maybe there will be one or two that you don't like at all, or an absolute favorite with the first sniff.

Which one was the first one that you smelled that made you decide to buy your oils? Was it the experience or was it the promise of the health benefits that attracted you first?

This is the time to just get to know your oils and become familiar with them!

When I began really using my oils, my daughter would come into my room every now and then, and open the box, put her face close to all of the bottles, and just inhale deeply. It was something new to her – new to us all! We were entranced!

2) Line Them up in Pretty Little Rows

Next, it is fun to take all of your little bottles of oils out, put labels on them and get them organized and available to use. Line them up. Look at the labels on each bottle. I think that they are beautiful and I love to look at the colors and the names of the oil on each of the labels! Notice that some will have supplement facts on the bottles. (This is your clue about which ones can be used internally as those without the supplement facts should not be ingested. A supplement label indicates that an essential oils has been approved by the U.S. Department of Food and Drug Administration to be Generally Recognized As Safe – or GRAS – for human consumption).

You have a box and stickers – that's good! Start by putting label stickers on the lids and organizing the bottles so that you can find what you want quickly when needed. If you don't have a box or stickers, make your own until you do. When I started, I took neon colored square garage sale stickers and a marker, and cut them to fit. I found a small cardboard box and put them there in alphabetical order.

Now I have a large box in my bedroom, a small box in the kitchen and a small rack in the bathroom, plus a makeup case in my purse for those I will need on the go! I used to have a purple zippered key fob with eight 5/8 dram bottles that I filled with my most commonly needed essential oils to take with me.

(NOTE: I've shared so many of the samples and small zippered keychain cases that now I just keep larger, 5 ml, bottles with me and take empty 5/8 dram bottles in case I need to fill them and give them away. I decided to save myself a step! Once you begin using essential oils, you get so excited about them that you tend to want to share them with others who can benefit from them as well.)

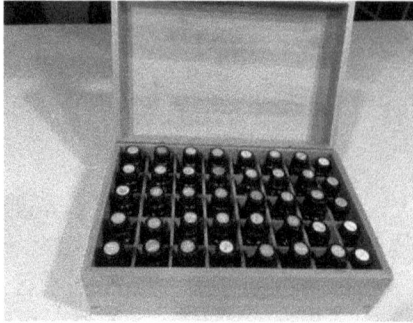

Some people line up their bottles in alphabetical order inside a box. Others organize them by color. Still others put those they use most close at hand. Just do it in a way that works for you because they are YOUR oils and are for you to use and find quickly and easily.

Even with a small box, you have room for more oils. You may wonder how you will ever fill it up! Or if you would ever really need to! If you begin with a kit of 10 or 20 oils, it seems like a lot and as though you have everything that you could possibly need. As you begin to really use them, likely you will find that they work for you for a variety of health concerns. You will find more and more things that they can be used for so you will likely quickly fill up your box.

3) Keep Them Close at Hand

Keep your oils somewhere handy. In order to find out how they can help you, they need to be close by so that you can try them out readily and easily.

You need to see them and remember that you have them! If they are not where you will think about using them, and quickly available, they will stay in the bottle, looking neat and pretty, but not doing you much good. Sound silly?

I can't tell you how often this actually happens…including with myself! When I began my journey in using essential oils, I found a couple that I liked, but didn't know what to do with most of my oils. I had a book about them, but the first time that I opened the book, my eyes glazed over – and I have a doctorate degree! I thought to myself, "Well, some day I will read through all of this, but not now!"

Believe me, however, once you catch on, you will want them with you at all times. Remember that zippered key case I was talking about? Many people find that these come in very handy.

I remember early on looking up a couple of health conditions in my book and noticing that there were several oils listed for each health issue, several conditions listed for each oil, and it didn't seem at all easy to keep straight, as to which supported what, or what to use and when. I was confused! Plus, I was busy!

So, I put the book with the oils, away in a cupboard, and didn't open more than the few that had familiar names. I figured I would get to it – when I had more time. It was about 8 months later that I put the box on my dresser and really began to delve into the prize that I had at my fingertips! I really wanted to know what essential oils were all about! I read the book from cover to cover – finally!

I wasted a lot of time, not knowing, and not doing anything with my oils. My hope is that by giving you this guide, you won't wait so long and will benefit sooner!

4) Keep A User's Guide Handy

Even though it may seem overwhelming in the beginning to open up a book listing and discussing essential oils, having a good reference guide is a must and something that even after a couple of years, I still go to often. In fact, I have several guides and more than one copy of my favorite that is now tabbed so that I can look things up easily. I keep one at my office, one in my home office and one in my kitchen. I even keep a small guide in my purse with my small bottles of oil samples.

I also keep an online resource open or as a favorite in my phone and so that it is easily accessible when I need information. The more you go to these various resources, the more you will learn and remember. It will get so that you are just confirming what you think is needed intuitively, just like you learned about other health and wellness practices throughout your life.

Look things up for yourself and then begin looking them up for other people. Aim to become familiar with how to find essential oil information quickly. You never know when an emergency will arise and when you need to know something quickly!

Recently, I was traveling and burned my hand badly with hot water from the coffee maker. I grabbed my lavender and began rubbing it over the affected fingers and part of my hand, including around a ring that had become so hot, it kept burning my skin underneath it! I had visions of having to deal with the pain of that burn all day throughout the conference, taking away from my ability to enjoy it. But no! I was pleasantly surprised when, after a few minutes, the pain was gone and there was absolutely no redness anywhere on my hand whatsoever! Had I traveled without my oils, it could have turned out quite differently! (I am also always prepared to call my doctors or other healthcare providers when needed and recognize that each practice, traditional and complementary, has its role in my healthcare.)

5) Don't be Afraid to USE Them!

In the beginning we can all feel overwhelmed not knowing what to do with our essential oils or how to use or apply them. Hopefully this guide will be helpful in getting you started.

Some people hesitate to use their essential oils because they don't want to waste them. Every drop is precious! While I do agree that every drop is precious, I think in terms of what they can do for my body and health. My body and my health are also precious! I imagine how they can help me!

One issue for some initially may be the cost. It can seem like a lot of money to buy an entire set of essential oils all at once!

However, when you really think about it, and that only a drop or two is needed at a time, then you consider how many drops are in a bottle of essential oil, you get a better idea of the true cost. Many essential oils come in 5 ml or 15 ml bottles. There are approximately 85 drops in a 5 ml bottle and around 225 – 250 drops in a 15 ml bottle. Doing a little calculating, you will begin to see that using essential oils is actually very cost effective and will ultimately save you money.

Not only do you use very small amounts, commonly 1 – 3 drops, if you are healthier in the long run, you will spend much less on your total healthcare during your lifetime. Additionally, essential oils last years in a cool, dark place maintaining their freshness and effectiveness. The main thing to keep them fresh is to keep them away from heat. I never leave mine in the car, for example, or out in the sun.

Because essential oils adapt to the body's needs, one oil or blend will be useful for a variety of complaints based on the body system rather than needing something specific to support a specific health concern. Digestive issues are a case in point. Typically, we might do something different for diarrhea, constipation, motion sickness, flu, nausea, vomiting, or heartburn. With a digestive blend of essential oils, the body can be supported in bringing itself back into a healthy balance with most digestive needs and would cost less than $.15 per drop! How much do our other options cost? Even if we need to integrate with other options, we may find that regaining our body's equilibrium will come more quickly when we add in our essential oils.

6) Daily Use versus Being Prepared for Emergencies

Just as many of us take supplements daily, there are some essential oils that are good to use on a daily basis as a means of helping our body ward off the negative effects from the environment such as toxins in the air, our carpets, exhaust, and even from other people who may be ill and carrying bacteria and/or viruses around with them.

We have to face it! No matter how much we do to protect ourselves by eating healthy foods, avoiding processed, hormone or pesticide-laden foods, and fast foods, we are exposed to a great deal in our air that we can't avoid completely.

We have the option to take our protection up a notch now! We can use a variety of essential oils on a daily basis, rather than only waiting to use them when that emergency situation arises.

It's good to be prepared for emergencies and know which essential oils to use, but consider what it will mean to your overall health if you just don't get sick as often, or as severely, or you reduce the number of sick days you take, or you have more energy to do the things you want to do in your life! We can't put a price tag on these things!

So, as you review the topics in the next few chapters, and the chapter where other essential oils users share their experiences, consider how you will want to fit this new complement to your health into your daily life, as well as learning what you need to know so that you, too, will be well prepared for the common health concerns when they arise.

7) What to Expect

While many have publicized and we hear stories about healing and miraculous changes, it is important to have a good understanding of how our bodies work, the role of medical professionals, our own responsibility in the matter, and where exactly essential oils fit into the picture.

Essential oils do not prevent, treat or cure disease. As we have all been told all of our lives, what we do, how we live, and the lifestyle choices that we make are what will either prevent disease or not. Genetics also play a role in our body's ability to ward of pathogens and disease processes, but they are not the final answer.

Our doctors and medical professionals are there to treat the symptoms of disease and illness, and to set broken broken bones, for example, or other more major problems. They can give us medications and provide other interventions, but they don't prevent disease and they don't cure us from diseases. Medications don't actually cure us, either, or they would work all of the time on every person for every disease!

What cures us is our own body! YES! It is a marvelous machine and does a great job most of the time, when we help it along, in healing disease and sicknesses, body injuries and other problems.

So, what is our responsibility in all of this? We can't change our genetics, and we can't avoid being exposed to many environmental toxins that are out there, but we can learn how to support and help our body resist disease and heal itself when it is experiencing problems.

This means that we can't expect to do things that we know cause harm and expect our body to stay healthy – no matter how many oils we spread all over us! We can't exist on Twinkies and Coke and expect to have energy, stay healthy, and not get cavities! We can't load up on sugar and food that contains minimal nutrients and expect our body to make good use of something we don't give it. We have to give it the raw materials! Our body has to have something to work with.

Imagine a king presiding over a kingdom. If his subjects are all sick or die, who does he have to ask to do the work around the land? If he doesn't give them food and keep them healthy, they will be worthless in keeping the kingdom moving smoothly.

When we take care of our bodies by giving it good nutrients, exercise, and adequate sleep, we are well on our way to having healthy cells and organs and more like the king of a flourishing kingdom.

Further, if we can reduce stress by working on our thoughts, having healthy, happy relationships, jobs that we enjoy, and a sense of purpose in life or spirituality, these are also things that will contribute to our body being able to heal itself.

It does us no good to brood over the things we cannot change, but does us a great deal of good to recognize where WE can make good choices.

Our essential oils are a wonderful addition to any wellness program!

3 WHAT TO DO NEXT: THE A, B, C'S OF USING ESSENTIAL OILS

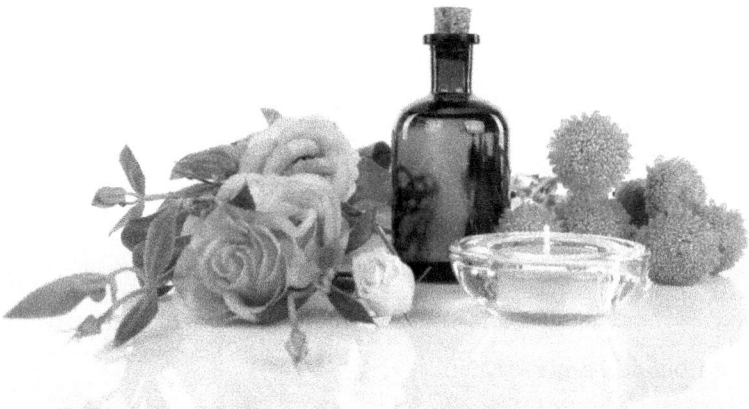

A: *Applying Essential Oils*

The first guideline about applying essential oils is to apply them as soon as possible after first noticing symptoms or being injured, for the best support for your body. Also part of the first step is recognizing the need to contact a healthcare professional with anything other than commonplace issues.

The next rule of thumb is to apply as frequently as every five minutes when an illness is severe, even if on the way to the doctor, or when a condition is progressing or getting worse. Apply two to four times a day if you catch something early, or one to three times for ongoing or chronic conditions.

The amount to use will depend upon body size with only one to five drops diluted, on average, for children or pets and up to twice that much or more for adults.

There is no one true right way that everyone should replicate when using or applying essential oils. There are many opinions about it, however. Some say that essential oils should only be used aromatically. "Aromatherapy" ("Aromatherapie") was the term coined by a French chemist named Rene-Maurice Gattefosse to describe the use of essential oils. Even the name implies that it is the aroma that induces the therapeutic benefit.

However, what we have learned since those earlier days of essential oil use is that using more than one method of application can actually improve the outcome. Sometimes using more than one essential oil will create a more profound or synergistic effect.

In Europe, the various countries had differing beliefs and preferences about how essential oils should be used. For example, the English favored topical use, the French favored topical and internal use, while the German's focus was on the inhalation or aromatic benefits of essential oils.

Some people feel better using essential oils topically. I once heard a speaker say that because each essential oil has many beneficial uses, if you didn't know what to do, you could pretty much simply close your eyes, reach out and grab one, and dump some of it on your head! He said that we make it much more complicated than it needs to be. Maybe so, but it still feels safer to know what to do.

The third method of use is taking them internally. There has been information online telling us that we should never ingest essential oils. But what is the problem? They come from plants and we eat plants! We feel fine about putting chemicals in our mouths when a doctor tells us to yet the idea of putting the extract from a plant into our mouths somehow is difficult for some to consider! There IS reason for some education and caution, however.

There are a few essential oils that are not appropriate to ingest, so do some investigating prior to jumping in with both feet on internal use. One issue with internal consumption of essential oils has to do with the manner in which they are processed. Look for oils that don't use chemicals in the extraction process. Other reasons have to do with some of the compounds found in the actual essential oil itself.

Essential oils are very, very potent – some studies say that they are up to 50 to 70 times as potent as the herbal form of the plant. As an example, a drop of peppermint essential oil is said to have the same potency as 28 cups of peppermint tea! (And this is an excellent example of how to use essential oils internally!) So, whichever method feels best to you, remember that a small amount goes a long, long way!

What is your feeling about it? We each have our own preferences!

The following is a review of the various application methods of essential oils in more detail:

1) Aromatic or Inhalation.

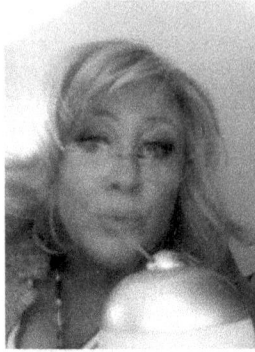

This method is by far the quickest pathway. It is also a good way to begin the use of essential oils in simple and effective ways. We can accomplish this with use of:

~ Diffuser: puts a fine mist into the air for inhalation and to freshen and improve air quality. Can last for hours in the air. It is best to use a diffusion method not involving heat, which can alter the therapeutic properties of the oils.

~ Direct Inhalation: by putting a drop of oil into our hands, rubbing them together, and then inhaling while cupping our hands over our mouths OR simply open the bottle and inhale!

~ Hot Water Vapor: add a drop to warm water in a bowl or sink, put a towel over the head while bending over the bowl or sink.

~ Fan or Vent: Put oil on a cotton ball and place in fan or vent, such as in the car or an office.

~ Perfume: Apply 1 or 2 drops to neck or wrists for the aroma, as well as topical support. (OR, create a perfume by adding to alcohol and distilled water.)

~ Cloth or Tissue: Put 1 – 2 drops on cloth, paper towel, tissue, cotton ball, handkerchief or spray in diluted form on pillowcases and sheets and inhale. If on a cotton ball or other cloth, keep in a baggie for later use.

How long to diffuse?

TIP: Diffuse for 15 minutes on, then 45 minutes off.

It has been found to be best to diffuse for 15 - 20 minutes per hour rather than to have a diffuser going constantly. This gives the olfactory system time to recover prior to receiving more oils and their compounds. Several times a day is good, or even 15 minutes on and 45 minutes off all day, which can be accomplished by using a timer if you have one available.

2) Topically

Topical application includes placing oils on the skin, hair, nails, or even in the mouth or on the teeth (still considered topical because they would be expectorated or "spit out" after as in "oil pulling"). When applying directly to the skin, remember to rub in for a few seconds before the essential oil evaporates. There will not be the usual oily residue you might expect from a typical "oil."

TIP: Start with a carrier oil to dilute the essential oil when beginning topical application for the first time and with any new (to you) essential oil.

The simplest and safest rule of thumb for topical application when you are just beginning to use essential oils, or with a person who doesn't know if their skin will be sensitive to them or not, is to start with a "carrier oil" and dilute the essential oil that you have selected. You can do that by simply applying the carrier oil first onto the skin and then applying the essential oil, or you can mix them together in a glass container or rollerball and then apply.

A "carrier oil" is simply an oil that is neutral, and that can act as a base for the essential oil. It will not dilute the effectiveness and in fact can help the effect of the essential oil last longer. It is called a "carrier oil" because it carries the oil onto the skin. Examples of "carrier oils" are olive, almond, avocado, coconut, and jojoba oils. Carrier oils as used topically are commonly derived from plants and have either no scent to a nutty, sweet scent. If they smell strong or have an unpleasant odor, they may be rancid and best not used. Fractionated coconut oil is preferred due to its own health benefits and long shelf life.

Methods of topical application:

~ Neat: Many oils can be applied "neat" or undiluted to the skin. Take care and be cautious with each new oil you use on your skin to be sure. For anyone with sensitive skin, or with children, or older adults, or weak immune systems, be especially cautious and always dilute with a carrier oil, or neutral lotion first.

~ Diluted: Diluting is the process of adding small amounts of an essential oil to a carrier oil to minimize the risk of a reaction to those with sensitive skin, babies, elderly, or those with compromised or weak immune systems. Another indication for dilution is with a "hot" oil. Examples of "hot" oils are: oregano, cinnamon, cassia and thyme.

~Massage: For massage, a couple of drops can be added to a neutral massage oil. You can ask the massage therapist to add some oils that you like when you get a massage. When I get a pedicure, for example, I take my essential oils with me and ask them to add a drop or two when they massage my feet and calves. Sometimes I have even "tipped" them with an essential oil if they enjoy them as much as I do!

~Shower: In the shower, oils can be used topically by adding a couple of drops to a washcloth or sponge or with a neutral shower gel to be

rubbed into the skin for additional health benefits when cleansing and to rub in afterwards. (Note: A few drops can be added to a bath [see below] or directly to the shower floor after turning on the water for an aromatic experience.)

~ Hair: There are prepared shampoos that contain essential oils or essential oils can be added into your shampoo or used after rinsing your hair.

~Compresses: To create a compress, simply fill a sink basin with hot or cold water, add a few drops of the desired essential oil, stir vigorously, and then lay a hand towel on the top of the water. Wring out the towel and apply to desired area.

~Bath: Add 3 – 6 drops to bath water. Start with a smaller amount as the skin will quickly absorb the oils that will be on the surface of the water.

~Body spray: To create a body spray, dilute a few drops of essential oil with distilled water in a spray bottle. There are a few reasons why someone would do this. Some will carry a spray with a citrus oil for cleaning their hands as with a hand sanitizer. Others will use an oil for calming and spritz when they feel stressed. Still others will use a favorite essential oil for its aroma as with a perfume. (For actual perfumes, alcohol is often used and there are specific recipes and processes for the creation of actual perfumes as we know them. For beginners, if the aroma is desired, many simply apply their favorite essential oil either neat or diluted to the area behind their ears and on the insides of their wrists.)

~Rollerball: For simple application topically, many people like to create rollerballs. Children especially like rollerballs because they are able to apply the oils by themselves. Empty rollerballs can be ordered through a variety of companies.

To create a rollerball, simply dilute a few drops of essential oil, or a blend of essential oils, with carrier oil, snap the roller piece into place, put on the lid and shake to blend.

How much should I use?

Usually just a drop or two is good. Some specific protocols may suggest other amounts, but in general, remember that a little bit of essential oil, with consistent and frequent use is better than using a large amount at one time.

TIP: A little bit, with frequent, consistent use is better than a one-time dousing in an essential oil. In fact, using more sometimes reduces its effectiveness!

Where do we apply essential oils?

When considering where to apply essential oils, we have many options. One option, for general use or if you are unsure of how the person will react, is to apply the essential oil to the bottoms of the feet, back of neck or pulse points (wrists and behind ears). For general purposes, such as simply wanting to support the body without a specific issue in mind, bottoms of the feet is a good place to begin. Some use this placement when they are seeking grounding or protection against environmental threats. Another time to consider the bottoms of the feet for placement is when there could be sensitivity, or with children. It is still a good idea to add a carrier oil to the bottoms of the feet first and then apply the oil or blend that you have selected.

When your purpose is to support your mental and emotional health, application around the chest, neck or shoulders is good. The back of the neck is an excellent location and where many will apply frankincense, for example, or a grounding blend. If you wish to have both aromatic and topical benefits, applying to the upper chest or even around the nose can be helpful. I often do this with my orange essential oil, which is very helpful in creating a pleasant, uplifting experience.

When there is a specific area of discomfort or concern that we wish to support by using an essential oil, we can simply use common sense and apply to that region of the body. For anyone needing respiratory support, applying to chest or across the bridge of the nose can be helpful. For those experiencing digestive issues, the abdomen is a good choice. For general internal cleansing or detoxification, since the liver is often involved in removal of toxins from the body, rub the oil over the area on the right side of the belly where the liver is located.

When I apply my essential oils topically, I rub them into my skin very well (so that I get the full benefit and they don't simply evaporate into the air) and then make sure to wash at least my fingertips so that I don't inadvertently rub my eyes afterward!

To review, here are the basic tips for *where* to apply essential oils:

- *General Use:* For quickest application and best absorption, apply to the bottoms of the feet, where pores are larger making absorption quicker, or over pulse points of wrist and behind ears.
- *Brain and Mood Support:* The back of the neck is another common application site for anything related to the brain, mood, or emotional support.
- *Specific Issues:* When deciding where on the body to apply the oil, think of why you selected it and place it on or near that part of the body.

The important thing is to apply!

Essential oils are wonderful in their ability to travel to where they are needed and support parts of the body where they can be useful.

* Caution: Take care not to touch or rub around the eyes with hands that have been touching essential oils!

2) Internally

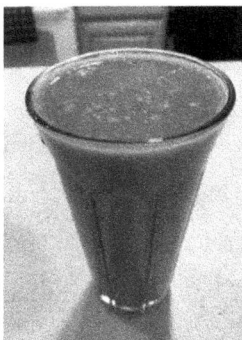

How do I know if an essential oil can be consumed or taken internally?

You will likely be told or find somewhere on the internet, or have a family or well meaning friend tell you that essential oils should NEVER be taken internally! My son-in-law came to me and challenged me about this practice after I had introduced one of the essential oil blends to the family, using it under our tongues. I had been told that this practice was fine with the oils I was using, and had had my own positive experiences but I was new and unsure so I did some research – I certainly didn't want to harm anyone! The fact of the matter is that truly depends. I thank my son-in-law for his concern and for making me learn more about it. The truth is that an essential oil or blend *can* be ingested if it meets certain criteria:

~ It must be pure and from a trusted source.

~ If there is a supplement label on the bottle, and it has been determined to be GRAS, or "generally safe for consumption."

~ If it is part of a blend that has a supplement label on the bottle.

If in doubt, or if you are just unsure about how you personally will respond, if you are not comfortable or squeamish about internal consumption, or if you just don't like the taste, you can always use the aromatic or topical methods instead.

There are many oils that can safely be consumed internally. Remember that this will depend upon the way that they are processed as well as the specific oil being selected. So, do your homework first! Check with the manufacturer of the brand you have, and ask about their methods of processing, standards and testing used, and look at the bottle itself.

Once you have determined that the oils you intend to ingest are appropriate for this type of use, the following are the most common methods for internal use:

~Sublingual: A couple of drops under the tongue is a quick and effective method.

~Roof of mouth: Place a drop on the thumb and rub on roof of mouth for quick absorption.

~ Capsules: Empty gel capsules can be purchased and filled with a few drops of an essential oil or a variety of them and then swallowed. For those who don't like the taste of a particular oil, but who want to ingest them, this is a good method.

~ Beverages: Essential oils can be added to water, tea, smoothies, or other beverages. EX: a drop of peppermint can be added to hot chocolate for a chocolate mint drink! Many simply enjoy adding a drop or two to their drinking water.

~Cooking: Essential oils can be added to cooking and baking, remembering to only use a drop or two. Even dipping a toothpick into the oil and then stirring into the food will add a great deal of flavor. There are many recipes available when you do a simple "google" search.

Be open to discovering the method or methods that seem best for you, your family and lifestyle.

B: Begin YOUR Journey

This IS a journey! And it can be a lot of fun. Begin your journey in the use of essential oils slowly so that you don't get overwhelmed. One suggestion is to select one essential oil that you like the smell of or that meets a particular need for you and begin there. If you really like a couple, then learn about them. Go to the resource of your choice (book or website) and look up the oils that appeal to you.

I would love to suggest that any user of essential oils take the time to learn about them. Learn about the plants themselves, and even which part of the plant (seeds, stem, leaves, bark, etc.) is used for your specific essential oil. I love the feeling of becoming connected to these plants! I love the sense of connection to the earth that I feel when I know more about the plants and what is required to obtain the oils. I love learning about where in the world they have been harvested and about the communities that grow the plants! Often there is tradition that is passed on from generation to generation. There is something special about knowing about those who have spent their lives caring for the plants and harvesting them that is unifying to us all! When I understand the process required to obtain my small bottle of essential oil, it takes on much deeper meaning for me. I strongly suggest that anyone using essential oils take the time to search for videos or articles about the harvesting and the process required. It is a humbling experience!

Consider the various methods of application for the particular oil you have selected and your particular need and begin to experiment. Be in the moment and see how you feel when you smell and apply it. How does it make you feel, both physically and emotionally? Do you notice anything? Some people notice the smell, others notice a physical or an emotional reaction to the smell or to the oil itself.

Once you have investigated the oils that appeal most, take a minute to consider those that you don't like. Some theorize that even an instant negative reaction to an oil might indicate that this is one that we may need for some reason. Once we smell an essential oil, it is already having a reaction in our body. Could it be that the toxin it could help to remove may want to stay there and sends a message to us to stop? Just one theory!

Many people enjoy journaling and the journey to making essential oils part of a health and wellness program is a good time to do this. It helps to log the results you have so that you will remember which ones affect you in which ways. Our reaction can even change over time, depending upon what needs we have at a given moment.

The key is to not be afraid and to just begin with an oil and a method of delivery that feels comfortable.

Some common ways to begin are to use oils aromatically, diffusing them. If you have a diffuser, that is an easy way to begin. Select one essential oil, such as orange, lemon or peppermint for daytime, or lavender for nighttime. Only a few drops are needed with water in most ultrasonic diffusers. Of course, the simplest method is to open the bottle and smell though some experts say that there is a difference between smelling from a bottle and smelling on the skin or from a diffuser.

Another common way to begin is to add a drop of a pure essential oil to water, tea or a smoothie. Lemon, orange and peppermint are oils that are commonly used for internal consumption, but only if they are pure and from a trusted source. Remember that essential oils are extremely potent so a drop or two is all that is needed.

Others prefer topical use and may want to apply an essential oil to the skin – peppermint to back of neck for cooling, for example, or lavender for calming. As a beginner, dilute until you know your own skin and body and how you react.

This is YOUR journey. We often expect to have the same results as the next person. You will find that your experience is often unique to you.

When you look in most guides on essential oils, several oils are listed and can be used for the same health concern. It doesn't mean use them all, necessarily, though there may be times when you would want to, once you have become more accustomed to how they work on you personally. When several are listed, it simply means that they share a chemical component that is helpful for that specific health concern or has properties that have been shown in research to be effective. Start with one and see how it works, then try another and record your experiences. Soon you will find what works best for you, your family, and for your specific needs.

Are you ready to begin?

C: Consistency

It has been suggested by many experts that essential oils be used on a regular, consistent basis. Many of them can be used occasionally for specific health supporting benefits, while there are many that can be used on a regular basis for overall health and wellness.

With essential oil use, we may be surprised because we can often notice instant results. If we put peppermint on the back of the neck, for example, we will immediately feel its cooling effects. If we inhale it, the effect will also be immediate. We can feel immediately calmer, or feel immediate relief from a burn with lavender.

I was visiting my grandsons a couple of years ago and as I approached the front door of their house to knock, the moisture on the steps caused my feet to slip out from under me and I fell on both knees on the cement landing. Ouch!! Pain! And a little worry because I have osteoporosis. I was very new to essential oils, but did have a few with me. I didn't really know what to use, but I had helichrysum, had heard that it was "powerful" and so I tried that. I immediately felt the pain subside! I remember the feeling of (pleasant) surprise and shock because of the quick relief from the pain that had literally taken my breath away just a moment before. Remember that this was MY personal experience and each of us will have our own results. I share this simply to say that sometimes we will notice immediate relief or support while other times, more commonly, we will gradually recognize that our health issue has abated or slowly improved.

With some oils and for chronic conditions especially, long term, consistent daily use is best. So, be consistent! Use oils daily or multiple times daily, depending upon the need, on an ongoing, regular basis. Make them a part of a daily routine, or lifestyle, just as with exercise, meditation, or any other healthy practice.

Consistent use of essential oils for emotional issues, such as occasional sadness or excessive worry, can help support the waxing and waning of emotional symptoms. These recommendations are not intended to replace any recommendations or medications prescribed by your doctor, but can be a helpful resource to add to your daily routine and to support your body's abilities to achieve a healthier state.

As a psychotherapist, I hear regularly that medications alone are often not enough and do not eliminate these emotional episodes. It is commonly recognized that the best solution is to seek psychotherapy or counseling while taking psychotropic (for emotional or mental conditions) medications. In addition, it is good to learn that there are essential oils and oil blends that have been specifically formulated to help with the emotional dips and surges that most of us experience. These are good to have on hand because they can be uplifting, grounding, balancing, and/or calming, thereby helping the body to obtain a more comfortable emotional balance.

We tend to deal with the normal emotional dips and surges on an as needed basis. It is actually more helpful, according to experts, to apply essential oils regularly and consistently for improved emotional stability and health. Using essential oils along with the other coping skills and stress management techniques often learned in counseling, is a better method for optimal emotional health. As always, consult with your healthcare professionals seeking counseling when recommended.

Most of us encounter other people with emotional issues, even if we don't suffer from them ourselves. If you have ever entered a room where there has been an argument, you will notice that the emotional tension in a room can be almost tangible and "contagious." Who hasn't felt another person's sadness or anxiety from time to time? There is a saying that, "The strongest emotion wins!"

I commonly use essential oils for mood management. As clients enter my office, they often bring their strong emotions with them. In order for me to work with them effectively, it is important for me to manage my own reactions to these strong emotions so that we all end the session better than when it began! So, even if you don't have emotional issues, likely you will encounter others who do. Having your own essential oils available, or used prophylactically (preventatively, consistently) will help you to manage such situations in a healthier manner.

Whether there is an emotional issue, a physical issue, or we are simply aiming to improve our health and prevent disease, essential oils used on a consistent basis can dramatically improve our outcomes by the manner in which they support our body. Many of my family members and friends, myself included, have reported that they have experienced fewer colds, headaches, less heartburn and other common concerns since they have begun to implement regular, consistent use of their essential oils, indicating an improvement in the functioning of our immune systems.

D: Daily Use

It almost goes without repeating that the consistent use of essential oils is most likely going to be daily use. While some people simply want a supply of oils to have on hand for emergencies, consistent, daily use is advantageous. The advantages of daily use are innumerable, so why not take full advantage of the power we have at our fingertips!

There are toxins in our environment from which daily use can help to protect us by supporting our immune systems. Daily use can help us to freshen the air in our homes and offices. We can give our immune systems a boost so that our body is more prepared to handle cold or flu viruses, reduce stress, and induce relaxation with daily use of essential oils. Essential oils have also been shown to support cellular regeneration and restoration of health. These are all on of list of the recognized functions of essential oils.

What does Daily Use look like?

Daily use for many includes adding essential oils to the shower or bath, shampoo or conditioner, and to the bottoms of the feet before dressing. It can include diffusing essential oils in the air first thing in the morning and adding a drop to a smoothie, water or tea. Cinnamon can be added to oatmeal, for example! Some choose to take supplements daily that include essential oils.

Later in the day, some may use a grounding blend, chamomile or lavender on the back of the neck or wrists if their day becomes hectic. They may put a few drops of peppermint, frankincense and wild orange into their hands and inhale for an afternoon pick-me-up! Others may add lemon, orange, a protective blend or a metabolic blend to their water and drink throughout the day.

In the evening, more oils may be diffused in the home to freshen the air or protect from viruses, bacteria or other toxins in the environment.

For someone who needs to unwind, use oils for calming and relaxing in a shower, the diffuser, or in a spray on the sheets and pillowcases. Specific oils can help some to relax and to sleep more peacefully.

Everyone is different, so experiment!

(Refer to Chapter 4 for specific examples of how real people use their essential oils and essential oil products on a daily basis.)

E: Experiment and Educate Yourself

Make it a goal to learn about your essential oils and how they work for you personally. Start slowly so that you don't get overwhelmed, but learn a little bit on a regular basis – even daily if you can. As mentioned before, find one essential oil that you like the smell of or that meets a particular need and begin there.

Go to the resource of your choice (book or website) and look up the essential oil you have selected to learn about it. Watch videos, attend webinars, conferences or other places where you can increase your understanding and become more educated. It helps to listen to some resources again and again so that the information becomes second nature to you. As you learn, tell others. I remember when I learned that the best way to really learn something is to teach it to someone else! Learn, then teach!

Once you have done your initial research, consider how you personally will want to use your oils. Try different methods. As you use it each day, while applying, remind yourself of its attributes or *why* you are using it and enjoy the experience. BE in the moment! Imagine the essential oil particles going to work and helping your body as intended. I like the use of affirmations as I do anything that I hope will benefit my health. Use each application as a time to be mindful and in the moment. This practice alone will reduce your stress levels.

As an example of where to begin to learn about some of the basic essential oils, there are lists online of how they are used. I like to make my own lists including the things that matter to me the most.

There are videos available online or found on Youtube on most individual essential oils. There are also recipes galore for Do It Yourself options for many, many purposes using essential oils, as well as recipes for healthy and enjoyable foods and treats.

There are other wonderful sources - too many to name. Many essential oils users have blogs, or have written books outlining their suggestions, experiences and giving you options. You can also find the books written by the well know experts in the field. A "google" search will lead you to treasure troves of information. Much of this will be anecdotal, or word of mouth, information, while some is based on research. If you go to PubMed, NIH, or WebMD, you will also find many, many articles of research that has been done with specific essential oils or essential oil compounds, which you can read through to see what was learned from such studies.

F: *Frequency and Quantity (For Adults, Children, Babies, and Pets)*

Essential oil use will likely be different from other health practices we have implemented. We may meditate daily, using breathing techniques, take supplements, or practice mindfulness regularly, but not necessarily frequently. The frequency for essential oil use is different than most other practices. The quantity or dosage is different as well and usually a good rule of thumb to remember is: "less is best."

We are used to the idea that if some of something is good, more is better. We have been conditioned to think this way because of how our doctors manage our treatments. Remember that we are not treating diseases, rather we are giving our bodies something to help it obtain health in its best way.

With essential oils, there is a point at which the effectiveness declines when more is used. So, more is not necessarily better! The most common quantity to use is around 1 – 3 drops of the selected oil for most needs.

On the other hand, another common mistake is to think that we should use just a tiny, little bit of our essential oil once, without follow up, and think we should see a huge improvement. Then, discouraged, we may say that they didn't work on us! This is more likely about not understanding about the needed *frequency* of use.

Frequency will depend upon whether something is "acute" (new and strong) or "chronic" (around for awhile, or ongoing), just starting, or going away. With essential oils, the frequency depends upon the situation.

For something acute, the rule of thumb is to use small amounts several times, say every 5 – 20 minutes until we feel relief – usually in about an hour or less. Then follow up by using every few hours. Oils move quickly through the body going to where they are needed.

For something chronic, or ongoing, or preventative, the frequency is different. A good rule of thumb is to use small amounts consistently 2 – 4 times a day on an ongoing basis for a regular, ongoing concern.

To review, we can reapply after a few minutes for an acute concern, or something that is just coming on, whereas for something ongoing, we may apply or use the oils a couple to a few times a day.

Babies and Children

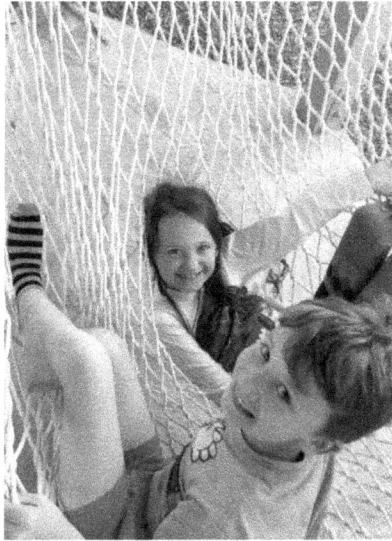

While children most often will not have negative reactions to essential oils, it is prudent to be cautious, just in case, and always dilute them.

- For babies under a year old, just one drop of essential oil diluted with about a teaspoon or up to a tablespoon of carrier oil is a good way to introduce them.
- For older children, 1-6 drops of an essential oil can be used per teaspoon of carrier oil, depending on the oil being used, the age of the child and their skin condition.

Diluting essential oils is a good rule of thumb for children and even adults at first until you see how someone will react to them. Remember –

they are potent!   And, diluting an essential oil does not reduce its effectiveness but rather allows for improved absorption and sustained benefit.

Pets and Animals

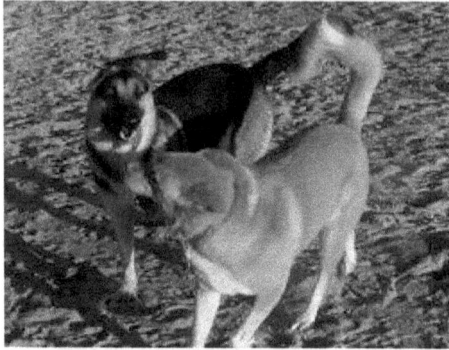

Many essential oils can be safely used with pets. There are precautions of which we should be aware, however. While many essential oils used on our pets are not only safe, but extremely effective, it is important to know about any adjustments we need to make and which oils to select, or avoid, for our specific breed of animal.

One veterinarian, Dr. Shelton, who uses essential oils with the animals in her practice, has done her own testing to be sure that they are not endangered or harmed. The urine and blood work done before and after exposure of the animals in her clinic has only given positive outcomes. Dr. Shelton became interested in using essential oils with animals when she found that the chemical air fresheners _did_ affect the animals' blood work!

Dilution is the first step to remember when using essential oils with our pets. It is important to dilute most essential oils when using them with pets. Often, the dilution is:

1 drop to 1 teaspoon, or up to 1 Tablespoon of carrier oil (Yes, similar to our children! Afterall, they are our fur-kids!)

A good way to accomplish this and to be prepared is to identify those oils you might wish to use regularly, obtain 5/8 dram sample vials, mix the carrier oil (FCO, fractionated coconut oil, recommended) with the specific essential oil, label and save for easy use. Consider it your Pet First Aid Kit!

Another option is to use rollerballs with the correct dilutions prepared ahead of time. For immediate use, simply cup your hand with the teaspoon of carrier oil in it, add your 1 drop of essential oil, mix together with your hands and apply to desired area. Yes, you will get some on yourself, but look at this as a side benefit! You may need to have someone hold your pet with this method, however. Alternatively, simply mix in a small glass cup and use a small amount, saving the excess for future applications.

Another general rule of thumb is to select diffusers for your home that combine the essential oils with water and provide a nice mist where pets are present.

Caution: Diffusers that pull straight from the bottle may not be ideal for pet households as the amount could be stronger than many pets' sensitive noses can tolerate!

Be sure that you are using pure essential oils not only for yourselves, but also for your pets.

Cats and Safe Essential Oils:

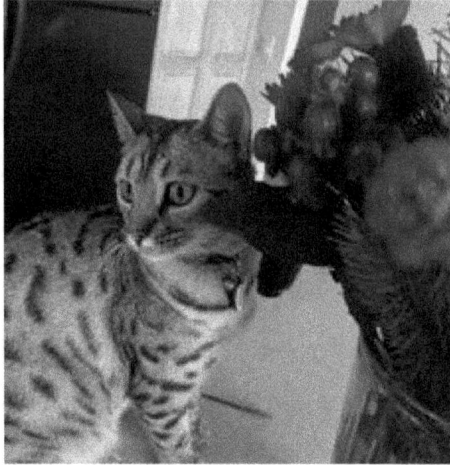

Use of essential oils around cats has many cat lovers upset and very, very cautious, and with good reason. They lack the liver enzyme glucoronyl transferase, which makes it difficult for them to metabolize some of the components in citrus essential oils and melaleuca (tea tree) essential oils. Dr. Shelton, DVM, has several cats herself and she was cautious as she began to use essential oils around them.

She monitored and tested for problems and began slowly. She noticed that one of her cats spent a lot of time close to the diffuser with lavender even delivering a litter of kittens right next to it. Ultimately, she came to the conclusion that the quality of the oils was what made the difference with how animals reacted, which is what we know about human use as well.

Good essential oils to have on hand for cats are:

Lavender, Frankincense, Helichrysum, Lemongrass, Cedarwood, Arborvitae, Cardamom, Eucalyptus, Marjoram, Sandalwood, Geranium,

Myrrh, as well as blends for digestion, calming, grounding, and blends to repel bugs and insects and protect from potential viral or bacterial threat

The oils to definitely keep away from cats are melaleuca and the citrus oils.

Treat cats like you would a child or infant and dilute the essential oils heavily (1 drop to 1 t. or T.) with a carrier oil such as fractionated coconut oil.

Remember, when diffusing essential oils with cats around, avoid using diffusers that pull directly from the bottle instead using those that mist with water and a few drops of oil.

Dogs and Essential Oils

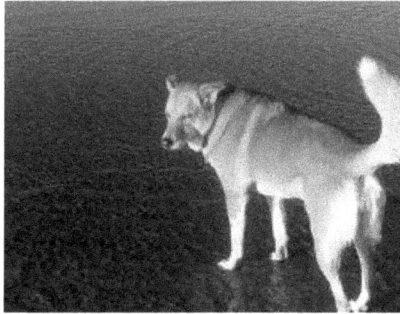

Dogs can also benefit greatly from the use of essential oils. Many have noted how their pet dogs can be calmed with lavender or how a dog's wound is helped in healing with frankincense or helichrysum.

Good essential oils to have on hand for use with dogs are:

Lavender, Frankincense, Peppermint, Helichrysum, Geranium, Lemongrass, Rosemary, Cilantro, Cedarwood, Cardamom and Arborvitae as well as blends for digestion, calming, grounding, to repel bugs and insects, and protect against viral or bacterial threats.

Other essential oils that are also safe to use for dogs are:

Basil, Bergamot, Roman Chamomile, Eucalyptus, Lemon, Marjoram, Clary Sage, Rosemary, Patchouli, or Sandalwood.

See Appendix C for a table of essential oils and their uses with dogs. Also, note the resources for pets in the reference section.

Other Animals

Whatever breed of pet you have, it is a good idea to do your homework prior to having an emergency where you would like to use essential oils. The resources listed in the reference section will help guide you and include uses for a variety of animals.

G: General versus Specific Use

Essential oils have been successfully used by most people who try them for general health and wellness. They can also be used for specific health concerns and benefits as they take on a supportive role for the body. Some oils have general uses, or can be used for a variety of purposes while others have more specific benefits. Most resources you will encounter list several oils for one health concern as well as listing the many that are supportive of general health and prevention of disease.

The thing to keep in mind is that the guidelines are just that – they are guidelines. We are all unique individuals and will find out by trial and error what works best for us for our desired purposes. The idea is to be open to trying a variety of oils and if one doesn't seem to work or we don't like how it feels for some reason, simply try something else.

Essential oils come from plants that have adapted to their environments, warding off pests and pestilences. If they have survived these enemies, they have properties that will help us to ward off bugs and diseases as well. We refer to them as being "adaptogenic." How this works for us is that inside our bodies, an essential oil that is good for digestion can be beneficial for all types of digestive issues. It is able to adapt to our specific digestive needs. In the long run, this will help us to cut costs after the initial outlay.

H: Household Use

Some people buy essential oils for the primary purpose of use in cleaning and disinfecting. They don't want to use toxic chemicals for cleaning and essential oils offer a "green" solution. Not only that, they work very well!

Oils that are commonly used for cleaning include lemon, wild orange, eucalyptus, peppermint, citronella (for bugs), rosemary, melaleuca (tea tree), thyme, lemongrass and white fir. They can be used with water, dissolved with a little alcohol before adding to water, added to a damp rag, or to the dishwasher before running it. For specific recipes, there are many blogs related to essential oils that list Do It Yourself recipes for many household purposes.

Some essential oils companies save you the trouble of creating your own cleaning products and carry a variety along with their line of essential oils. Some cleaning products available include hand cleansers, laundry detergent, and general household cleaning concentrates. Not only do they clean as intended, they have an added benefit of improving and freshening the air, reducing bacteria, viruses, fungus and mold, rather than adding toxins to our household environment.

If household use is where you choose to begin your essential oil journey, enjoy the results! Do stay open to other uses for your oils down the road as well! Make a journal listing each recipe that you try and before you know it, you will have your very own list of favorites!

I: *Internal Use*

There are many wonderful internal uses for essential oils. As a caution, once again, only pure essential oils from a trusted source should be taken internally. You will know if an essential oil can be taken internally if there are supplement facts on the label.

The internal use of essential oils is believed to originate from the French where a few drops of essential oils were added to honey, bread or vegetable oil and then consumed.

Some people will simply put a drop or two on or under their tongue. Others may want to ingest the oils but don't enjoy the taste so will put a couple of drops into empty gel caps and swallow them as they would any other supplement or capsule. (Empty gel caps can be ordered online or purchased at some local health food stores.) Other people will use essential oils in beverages such as water, tea or smoothies, or in baked goods. My favorite way to use them internally is in smoothies and teas as well as in my water.

As soon as you begin to put essential oils in your food or beverages, someone is likely to tell you that you shouldn't. Remember that not all oils are appropriate for ingestion so you do have to know your essential oils.

There is some justification for the concern about the safety of the internal consumption of essential oils. Besides the fact that some oils are not intended for internal consumption, there are companies that use processing methods where chemicals are involved which affect the safety of the oil making them unfit for ingestion.

When essential oils have been obtained through steam distillation or cold pressing, they are more likely fine for internal use, if they are pure. The problem lies when chemicals are used in the extraction process, or when other elements are added. There are oils that are touted as pure that might not meet the standards required for the safe ingestion of essential oils. Again, be sure that they are pure and approved for ingestion by their manufacturer. You would be wise to take it a step further and investigate the methods used for certifying the oils that you purchase prior to assuming that they will be safe. For more suggestions about internal methods of essential oil use, refer above to "A: Applying Essential Oils".

J: Journaling

Journaling was mentioned earlier as a recommended practice as you begin your journey in the use of essential oils. The reason for this is that it is important for you to remember your experience – what you like and what you don't like, how you used it, and what worked best for you. With so many options, it is easy to forget! No one is the same and no one person has the exact same experience with essential oils as another person. Sometimes there will be a combination that you come across that you prefer. Don't feel discouraged if something recommended by someone else doesn't give you the same experience. Consider it your own personal path and enjoy the process!

Many oils contain properties that are helpful for many purposes and body systems. For example, in my family many of us experience headaches, and even migraines. You will find that several oils are beneficial in relieving the tension and stress that can be associated with these headaches. When the stress and tension is reduced, the headache itself is less painful. This is one way in which the body is supported with essential oils. I like the smell of a couple of them while my sister prefers a different combination. I don't need to refer to a journal now, but in the beginning, it was very helpful as I experimented to see what was helpful and when.

Use any kind of journal or notebook, or even keep track on a smartphone. As you begin, write down the name of the essential oil, how much you used and how it affected you. Note how you feel about the odor and the method that you have chosen to use it. Track your frequency and dosage. At bedtime, you may even write down something that you have noticed about how your day went in general. Later on, you may make connections that you don't notice immediately. Writing down the little things can help you to recognize the differences that the use of essential oils has made in your life over time.

K: Ketones, etc.: A Little Chemistry Anyone?

Don't be frightened! We will keep this discussion as basic as possible. But aren't you just a little bit curious about why essential oils do what they do? What is it about them that makes them so powerful and gives them the ability to have the effects that they are shown to have? I think it is important to have a basic understanding of the chemistry behind essential oils because it helps us to realize that there are actual molecules – real, tangible pieces of matter – that are at work when we use our essential oils. They are not simply "snake oil," or "voovoo juice" (quoting my nephew). There is a reason, an actual chemical reason, behind the efficacy of essential oils.

A quick review of the chemistry of essential oils will demonstrate this. It may not be something that you will need to know about immediately, and maybe you don't want to know about it at all! Most of us run into people, with all of our excitement and enthusiasm, who say using essential oils is nonsense! Whether or not you ever want to get into the depths of the nitty gritty chemistry behind essential oils, my hope is that you will at least nod your head and recognize that there is an actual concrete reason - a science – demonstrating that essential oils do something. They are not simply magic, or like a placebo that works because our mind tells us it should.

With confidence, you can say, "No, they do work! They have chemical constituents that have specific abilities. And they don't have side effects because they come in the form created in nature." Whether or not you really want to understand or even read this, it is important to at least understand that there is real chemistry, or chemical components with active properties in essential oils.

Start here...

What do you know about chemistry? What is it? It is the study of matter and energy and the interactions between them. My first recollection and image of chemistry is of sitting in a lab with the element table on the wall – you know, where you see abbreviations like Na (Sodium), Cl

51

(Chloride), etc.

When we break essential oils down into these chemical constituents, or small active parts, there are two major categories. You've heard of hydrogen, carbon and oxygen, right? These are on the element charts such as the one described above. Well, one group of essential oils is made of primarily hydrocarbons (hydrogen and carbon) and the other group is the oxygenated compounds, or those that have oxygen atoms as well.

Hydrocarbons

The primary classes of hydrocarbons found in essential oils are called the terpenes and are classified based upon the number of "isoprene" units present. We are mainly concerned with the classes called monoterpenes and sesquiterpenes.

Monoterpenes are present in nearly all essential oils. They do many things related to getting rid of toxins. Some are antiseptic and antibacterial, while others are antifungal, antiviral, antihistaminic, antirheumatic, anticarcinogenic, stimulating and insecticidal, to name a few. Some examples of monoterpenes are pinene, camphene, myrcene, and limonene. Some monoterpene alcohols are linalool, citronellol, and geraniol.

Interestingly, it is easier to list those essential oils that do NOT contain monoterpenes to a significant degree than those that do. Monoterpenes are NOT found to a significant degree in: basil, birch, cassia, cinnamon, clary sage, close, geranium, sandalwood, vetiver, wintergreen and ylang ylang.

Sesquiterpenes are also found in great abundance in essential oils. These are antibacterial, anti-inflammatory, slightly antiseptic and sedative. The impressive thing about the sesquiterpenes are that they are capable of crossing the blood-brain barrier and are able to enter the brain tissue.

I remember when my oldest son was hospitalized with a brain abscess at 5 years of age. I learned then that a problem the doctors experienced was that the medications they had available were not able to cross the blood-brain barrier, complicating his situation, and their ability to get antibiotics to the abscess in the right frontal lobe of his brain. (We did eventually win this fight and he is now an adult with a family of his own. He uses essential oils daily, too!).

Sesquiterpenes are found as constituents in several oils including: ginger, myrrh, sandalwood, vetiver, ylang ylang, cinnamon, clary sage, close, cypress, white fir, frankincense, geranium, helichrysum, lavender, lemongrass, meleleuca, and peppermint.

Are you beginning to see why it is not as critical to be super precise about the oils that you select and use? The actions overlap quite a bit and many essential oils take on many roles and functions. Frankincense is an example of one that has been called the "King" of oils because it has so many chemical components, and so it is capable of taking on many different actions.

Oxygenated Compounds

The most common oxygenated compounds we may want to know about are the *alcohols, aldehydes, esters, ketones, oxides and phenols.*

Alcohols are known for being antibacterial, anti-infectious, and antiviral, as well as being stimulating and increasing blood circulation. They are mild and pleasant smelling.

Aldehydes are the components that give an essential oil its wonderful aroma. They are powerful and calming to emotions. Some are antimicrobial, antiviral and antiseptic as well. They can be aphrodisiacs, relieve emotional stress, reduce blood pressure, and dilate blood vessels.

Esters occur when an alcohol and an acid react chemically, and they are very volatile. Almost all essential oils have at least one or more. They are found in the mildest oils, and tend to be calming, soothing, sedative, relaxing and balancing. They are antimicrobial agents, antifungal and antispasmodic, and are balancing to the nervous system.

Ketones are known for their ability to stimulate cell regeneration, promote the formation of tissue and liquefy mucous so are good in support of respiratory issues, particularly upper respiratory complaints. They also promote healing. They can be toxic alone, or when isolated, but are not found alone in nature.

Oxides are derived from other compounds that have been exposed to oxygen. They act as expectorants and are mildly stimulating. One of the most common oxides, 1.8 cineole, is anti-inflammatory, and good for asthma and pain.

Phenols are a group of compounds that are some of the most powerful in their antibacterial, analgesic, disinfectant, anti-infectious, and antiseptic properties. They have sharp and powerful odors and can be irritating to the skin. They are stimulating to both the nervous and immune systems. Oils containing large amounts of phenols are best diluted rather than used "neat" and used for shorter periods of time. Examples of essential oils containing phenols are basil, birch, cinnamon, clove, fennel, melaleuca, oregano, peppermint, thyme, and wintergreen. Some of these are considered "hot" oils and can burn the skin, so be cautious when using them topically.

Other less common compounds found in essential oils are *lactones, coumarines,* and *furanoids.*

Lactones tend to be phototoxic. This means that a person using them could have a skin reaction when in the sun after using essential oils with lactones. They have anti-inflammatory, expectorant, antitumoral, and antispasmodic properties and are used for health support. *Coumarines* are a subcomponent of lactones.

Furanoids are primarily found in citrus fruits that are obtained through expression methods. They can be phototoxic because they amplify the wavelengths of UV rays. Interestingly, myrrh essential oil, which contains ten times the number of furanoids as many essential oils, has been found to be non-phototoxic.

Essential oils are a good example of how something that might be toxic on its own becomes non-toxic when found as it was created in nature. Myrrh is one of these examples. Another is cineole, a common oxide with significant expectorant properties, which when in isolation has been shown to be toxic, but when found in nature, it is not.

Common Chemical Compounds and Associated Essential Oils

The following are a few of the more common chemical compounds found in essential oils with brief explanations of what they do.

Limonene (monoterpene)

Found in lemon, lime, orange, grapefruit, and bergamot.

Good for healthy cleansing, healthy cellular function and support, promotes healthy inflammatory response, supports healthy cholesterol, helps to purify microbes and supports getting rid of harmful chemicals and damaged cells.

Eugenol (phenol)

Found in rosemary, thyme, close, nutmeg, cinnamon, and basil.

Good for protecting DNA, supports getting rid of free radicals, and helps to purify microbes by poking holes in the bacterial membrane of cells which is where viruses often hide.

Pinene (monoterpene)

Found in lemon, eucalyptus, margoram, juniper, thyme, lavender, mint, helichrysum, rosemary, geranium, pine and frankincense.

Good for keeping insects at bay, supports healthy inflammatory response, and helps cleanse or purify microbes.

Carvacrol (monoterpene phenol)

Found in oregano, thyme, rosemary, and marjoram.

Good for supporting healthy cellular function, cleansing, antioxidant and purifying.

Linalool (monoterpene alcohol)

Found in lavender, coriander, sweet basil, citrus and mint.

Good for supporting healthy inflammatory response, promotes relaxation, soothing and calming, supports increase of dopamine activity, and promotes decrease in discomfort.

Menthol (monoterpene alcohol)

Found in peppermint, and eucalyptus.

Good for cooling, digestive support, relaxation of smooth muscle, supports decreasing topical discomfort and promotes purification.

1,8 – Cineol (Eucalyptol) (oxide)

Found in eucalyptus, rosemary, basil, lemongrass, melaleuca, thyme, and ylang ylang.

Good for supporting elimination of mucus, supporting healthy purifying and cleansing, promoting healthy respiratory function, promoting healthy inflammatory response and promoting decrease in discomfort.

Bottom Line...

When thinking about chemistry and essential oils, simply remember that essential oils are powerful. They are powerful in small quantities. They function on a cellular level through the action of chemical compounds. Finally, they are supportive of many aspects of health, promoting the fighting of disease, supporting the body's inflammatory response, helping the body ward off the "bad guys", and in promoting healthy aging.

L: Layering

Layering is the preferred method of using more than one essential oil for topical therapeutic purposes. There are blends that are premixed by those understanding the chemical properties of the specific oils and should be used rather than for a novice to attempt to mix their own blends initially.

Layering includes applying one essential oil topically, rubbing it in and then applying another essential oil on top of it. There is no need to wait any length of time prior to applying the second or third oils as the oils are quickly absorbed. A carrier oil can also be used either first (preferred) or after for dilution (or upon finding that one is sensitive to that particular oil or blend). Oils can be layered on any part of the body, including bottoms of feet, back of neck, down the spine, on the chest, on inside of wrists, and behind the ears.

There are specific practices where several oils are layered in a specified order and in a specified manner for a therapeutic effect. These are often associated with an essential oil company. Individuals can become trained and certified in performing these therapeutic applications of essential oils. The intent of any of these techniques is to create balance and harmony physically, mentally and emotionally for the person to whom it is administered.

M: Massage

A certified massage therapist will use their skills for the purpose of stimulating muscle, skin and connective tissues and can add an essential oil to support healing, and promote balance and wellness. Depending upon whether stimulation, relaxation, soothing or immune support is needed, a massage therapist can determine which essential oil might be added to the massage treatment. If you wish to have essential oils added when you are receiving a massage, simply ask your massage therapist to include them as most practitioners don't mind adding your oils to the routine.

A massage therapist who is trained and certified can also incorporate the techniques referred to above for additional benefit to their clients.

If someone who is not trained wishes to make and use oils for massage for family or close friends only, it is recommended that they use light to medium pressure or strokes and avoid doing anything requiring knowledge of anatomy and physiology. Combining carrier oils with essential oils and applying to the skin with care can have pleasant to therapeutic benefits. Certification is required when using these modalities in any kind of business practice.

N: Nose and Olfactory System

The theory behind how essential oils work aromatically is related to the nose and olfactory system. When essential oils are inhaled, the olfactory system is stimulated and a signal is sent to the limbic system where emotions and memories are contained. There are specific receptors for specific odor molecules. It is believed that the proximity to the amygdala and limbic system are the reason for the often strong physiological and psychological responses that are evoked as hormones and neurotransmitters are released.

The interesting thing is that even if a person's sense of smell is impaired, as when suffering from a cold or respiratory problem, aromatic use of essential oils still seems to be highly efficacious in supporting the body. It is believed that the reason for this is that the particles from the oils enter the blood stream, boosting the immune system and balancing body systems with their many therapeutic benefits.

O: Oil Pulling

Do you want whiter teeth, and even clearer and brighter skin? Some experts believe that when you practice oil pulling, because you are pulling toxins out of your mouth and eliminating them from being ingested and passed around through your system, they can help not only your teeth but also your skin and complexion.

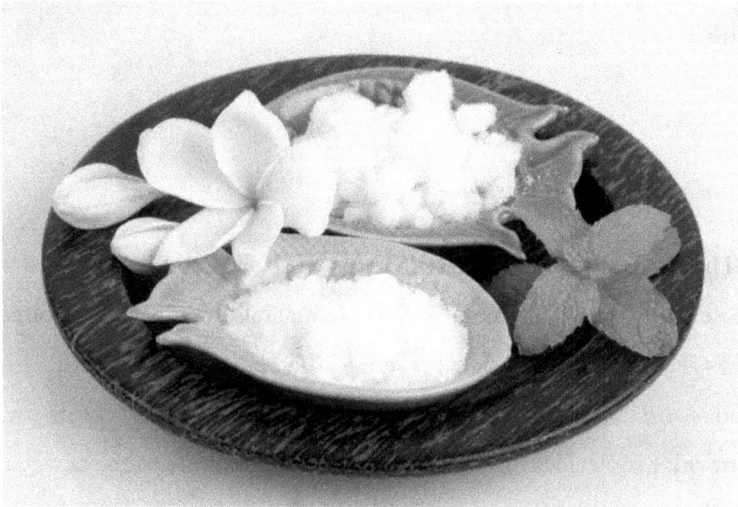

Oil pulling is a technique where a tablespoon of oil such as coconut, olive, grapeseed, or other high quality vegetable oil, is swished vigorously and "pulled" between and through the teeth for 5 up to 20 minutes and is then expectorated (spit out). A couple of drops of an essential oil can also be added. It is recommended to do this in the morning on an empty stomach and up to 3 times a day. It is important to spit out the oil as it will contain toxins and bacteria after the pulling. Oil pulling is considered a topical application of essential oils, since it is expectorated rather than ingested.

Some studies support oil pulling's efficacy in improving the health of gum tissue and mucous membranes in the mouth. It is also important to brush and floss, but the benefits of oil pulling have been shown to have many additional positive benefits to oral health. Interestingly, this procedure could have implications for prevention and treatment of many diseases by ridding the mouth of toxins and bacteria.

Among the dental community, the connection of gum disease (periodontitis) to heart health has long been recognized. More recently, connections have also been found between oral health and diabetes, stroke, and other health issues. Nearly half of all adults and many teens have some level of gum disease, so this is a concern that affects many of us.

Oil pulling has its roots in Ayurvedic medicine and gained popularity more recently (1990's) in Western culture. Some experts believe that it can be helpful for a long list of health concerns.

P: Purity and Potency

An essential oil's purity is its most important characteristic according to most experts. It is important to know about the purity your essential oils. Many people can tell the difference when they smell a pure essential oil that is potent and undiluted. Crucial to achieving and maintaining purity in essential oils are where they are grown, how they are grown and harvested, and how they are distilled. Additionally crucial is knowledge that they have not been adulterated in any way.

An essential oil that is pure should be free from pesticides, fillers, artificial contaminants, synthetic additives, or other chemical residues. We can trust oils that come from companies who do rigorous testing to determine chemical composition, potency and purity. Testing can also determine if an essential oil has been adulterated, or altered. Oils can be adulterated in a variety of ways, according to experts in essential oil testing and chemistry. Testing at various stages of growth and production and by third, objective parties, can give the most accurate results. Additionally, someone who knows how to read the tests and what each one indicates is required for accurate assessment.

Where a company sources their products is significant as it affects the potency. When a plant is grown under optimal conditions, the resulting oil will be of the highest quality and contain the highest amount of desired chemical constituents. We can grow pineapple in many parts of the world, but who will argue that they are sweeter when grown in Hawaii or other areas with the best weather and soil conditions. I remember eating corn and tomatoes grown in Illinois. I've had gardens where I have grown these vegetables as well, but I have yet to encounter the wonderful taste of those grown in the fields in the Midwest. It is the same with any plant. Since essential oils come from plants, it matters where in the world they are grown.

Be sure that you are getting oils from a trusted source, who researches locations around the world and finds the best conditions for the specific chemical constituents desired, and that they are free from pesticides and other contaminants or additives so that they have the purity and potency that your family deserves.

Q: Quality & Testing

What is the best process to be followed in the production of essential oils? First, the raw materials will be gathered from the ideal location. Next, they will be distilled or cold pressed, depending upon the plant. On sight, the resulting oil should then be tested using several tests that will indicate their purity, potency and if there are pesticides or other ingredients that should not be there. The kinds of tests that might be performed are:

- Organoleptic
- Gas chromatography
- Mass spectrometry
- Chiral GC testing
- Isotope Carbon 14 testing as needed

Next, the oil would be sent to the distributing company who would also test usually including:

- Organoleptic
- TPC/Microbial
- FTIR scan
- Specialized testing as needed

After passing these tests, the essential oils would be bottled and labeled. Finally, there would be a last evaluation prior to the oils being released for sale similar to the testing done before bottling. A bottle from each batch is saved in case it needs to be evaluated later on for something unforeseen.

Quality is related to purity and potency, as well as effectiveness. Essential oils are best when they are sourced from researched locations from around the world, where the soil and weather conditions are optimal, and where those conditions produce the chemical constituents in the best combinations for the specific purposes intended. Additionally, it is key that they and neighboring farms are free from impurities and pesticides.

The best, highest quality essential oils will stand up to the many types of testing done for purity and potency, including by third parties who have no ties to the company, and can give objective results. You want the company producing your oils to test them and give them their stamp of approval, after testing has been done and they are found to meet the required standards.

Be aware that any "stamp of approval" from an essential oils company is not the same as an FDA endorsement or designation. Companies that give high designations of purity are responsible to have integrity and to set and maintain a high standard. We deserve and need it for the health of our families.

It makes sense to pay attention to quality when selecting essential oils when you hope to achieve specific health benefits and outcomes. When we use potent, pure, high quality essential oils, they can be less expensive in the long run. Often, we can tell the difference when we open the bottle.

R: Reflex Points or Reflexology

The topical application of essential oils to specific points on the feet, hands and ears, that are believed to correspond to every organ and part of the body is called reflexology. Essential oils can be applied to both the reflex points and over the actual body part when support is needed there. Another time that reflex points can be utilized is when there is an area of concern, but skin sensitivity is an issue. In such cases, an essential oil can be applied on these points of hands, feet or even ears, with less risk of skin reactions.

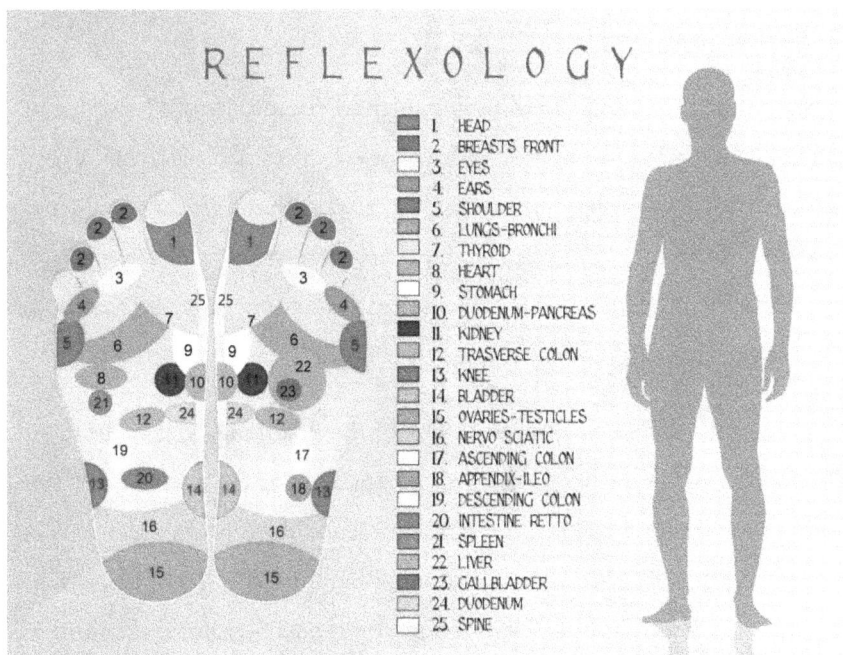

REFLEXOLOGY

1. HEAD
2. BREASTS FRONT
3. EYES
4. EARS
5. SHOULDER
6. LUNGS-BRONCHI
7. THYROID
8. HEART
9. STOMACH
10. DUODENUM-PANCREAS
11. KIDNEY
12. TRASVERSE COLON
13. KNEE
14. BLADDER
15. OVARIES-TESTICLES
16. NERVO SCIATIC
17. ASCENDING COLON
18. APPENDIX-ILEO
19. DESCENDING COLON
20. INTESTINE RETTO
21. SPLEEN
22. LIVER
23. GALLBLADDER
24. DUODENUM
25. SPINE

The practice of working on reflex points is an art and a science and many seek regular sessions with someone trained in reflexology for relaxation, balancing and a variety of other health benefits. A variety of research studies have been done on the benefits of regular reflexology treatments, including one with soldiers in Israel who found relief from PTSD (post traumatic stress disorder) symptoms. They experienced improved sleep, concentration and general improvement in their mood ('Reflexology on the Front Lines of Health Care', Massage Magazine, November/December 1998). The use of essential oils at home in conjunction with this practice increases the benefits they may provide. Meanwhile, as lay advocates in the use of essential oils, knowing that these are areas that can be of benefit in supporting specific body systems can serve as a guide in our determination of where to apply the oils at the very least.

S: Safety

Any time we bring a new healing method into our lives it is important to understand safety, along with efficacy or effectiveness. Safety involves being sure that one will be free from risk of injury, harm or danger. Many new users of essential oils wonder about their safety and can even be concerned that the methods that they try might have negative effects to themselves or their families.

Essential oils are very potent. One of the first things that we learn about them is that they are 50 – 70 times as potent as the plant or herb from which it is derived due to the concentration that occurs while distilling or pressing the oil. If you put one drop of lemon oil in a large glass of water, you will taste the potency! If you drip it on a Styrofoam cup, you will see the Styrofoam break down! While there are definitely times to be aware and cautious, pure essential oils that have passed tests of quality, purity and potency, and that are used as recommended by the company from whom they are produced, will be safe or have negligible risk.

"Although many essential oils are potentially hazardous materials, if handled in the appropriate manner, the risks involved in their use can be very small. So therefore, most commercially offered essential oils are safe to use for the purpose intended in a domestic/ professional or clinical environment" (Burfield, 2004).

What Factors Influence Essential Oil Safety?

The factors that influence essential oil safety are their quality, their chemical composition, how they are applied, the dosage and dilution, the integrity of the skin and the age of the person using the oil.

If an essential oil is pure, there is less likelihood that there will be an issue with safety. If an essential oil is adulterated, the likelihood of having an adverse reaction increases. Stick with pure, authentic, and genuine essential oils to be safe! (NAHA, 2014).

"Hot" oils, or those rich in aldehydes or phenols, are some that could cause a reaction to the skin and should be used with caution, diluting with topical application to be prudent. The most common "hot" oils are oregano, cinnamon, cassia, and thyme. Others that require some caution are clove, black pepper, peppermint and a protective blend, which contains several of these oils.

As the nickname "hot" implies, a reaction to the skin would occur right away if it were causing a reaction. Even though an essential oil is "hot" this does not mean that every person will experience a reaction to it. However, it is better to be safe and dilute "hot" oils or take them in a capsule internally.

A person's skin can become sensitized to certain oils, even if there is not a reaction initially. You would know if this is the case by the appearance of redness or blotchiness, sometimes accompanied by pain. If this occurs, the person may be sensitive to this oil for years* or indefinitely. Once again, it is better to be cautious and dilute rather than risk becoming sensitized to essential oils. (*Staying away from the specific oil causing the reaction for a lengthy period of time, such as 6 months to a year, and then retesting a diluted sample will determine if the sensitivity has become permanent or if the oil can be reintroduced in its diluted form.)

Each method of application of essential oils has safety issues, which should be considered. As noted, topical application can cause a skin reaction if the oil is "hot" or caustic. *The solution is dilution!* Inhalation carries a very low level of risk to most people and even animals due to the low concentration that might be carried in the air even with 100% evaporation. For internal use, when oils are pure, and from a trusted source, there is minimal safety risk when using small amounts in the manner suggested. These are areas that continue to be researched and evaluated.

When essential oils are used sparingly, which is what is recommended, and diluted as indicated, there is little concern for danger or harm. If skin is damaged, diseased or inflamed, it is more permeable to essential oils and may be more sensitive. Dilution is once again recommended in such cases.

Young children, infants and toddlers are more sensitive and just as they need differing amounts of food or other nutrients, so would the amount of essential oil recommended be different and in this case, less. Again, dilution is a good rule of thumb for babies and younger children. Since older individuals can have more skin sensitivities, a reduced concentration is indicated for this population as well.

Photosensitivity can be another concern. This is where the application of an essential oil could cause a reaction to the skin when the person goes out into the sun afterward. Bergamot is an essential oil that has been shown to demonstrate this reaction, along with other citrus oils that have been obtained through distillation rather than cold pressing methods.

Commonsense would tell you that you would not use an entire bottle of an essential oil at once. Learning about each essential oil as you use it, along with how, when and in what quantity to use it is the appropriate method. If you have questions, call the information line for the essential oil company and they are usually happy to help you with additional resources.

Not Recommended for Use in the Eyes

While there have been some reports of the use of essential oils being used in the eyes, unless being administered by a medical professional, such as a naturopathic doctor, keep essential oils out of your eyes. At the very least, they can sting and be uncomfortable, to causing a burn on the surface of the eye. If an essential oil accidentally gets into your eye, dilute with a carrier oil right away. (Note: Even severe burns have been reported to heal within a week or so (NAHA, 2014, Safety Information).

General Precautions for Safety

~ Keep essential oils out of the reach of children and animals.

~ Check for photosensitive oils and avoid prior to sunbathing or tanning.

~ Learn about the oils you use, and recommended uses and dilutions before using them.

~ Avoid the use of undiluted essential oils, especially when first using them.

~ Keep essential oils away from the eyes

~ Keep away from candles, cigarettes, matches and flames – they are flammable.

~ Use glass containers with essential oils, or plastics that have been specially formulated to contain essential oils, as they can break down plastics and Styrofoam.

For further information on the safety of essential oils, check out articles by the NAHA, National Association for Holistic Aromatherapy. www.naha.org.

T: *Topical Use & Beginnings of Aromatherapy*

Our knowledge about essential oils and their history over the centuries begins in Egypt and China where they were used for their aroma and for healing. The Greeks and Romans are also known to have used essential oils as aromatics. We know about Israel's use of aromatics and ointments from the New Testament. The Arabs are credited for steam distillation. Once the process of distillation was invented, Europe became involved in distilling essential oils as well and using them for perfumes.

During the Great Plague, it was found that those who had the most contact with aromatics, such as perfumers and spice traders, were seemingly immune to the plague while so many others died around them. This led to medicinal uses of essential oils by physicians. The French came on the scene in the 19th century using oils for their fragrances. The research they did led to the recognition again of the health benefits of essential oils. Finally therapeutic grade oils and knowledge about them became available again for public use.

The topical application of essential oils was primarily an English practice where tiny amounts of essential oils were diluted in a vegetable oil base (usually at a 1-3% concentration), and then the primary method was to massage the body with the diluted oil to produce a relaxing effect and relieve stress.

TIP: Take care to keep hands away from eyes whenever touching essential oils.

For more information about the topical application of essential oils, refer above to "A: Applying Essential Oils," under "Topical."

U: Uses Found in Research of the Chemical Components of Essential Oils

Essential oils have been found, through research and the study of the chemical composition and actions of each component, to have many uses and benefits for health and wellness. Various essential oils have been found to have some of the following properties depending upon their specific chemical composition:

Analgesic	Aphrodisiac
Anesthetic	Calming
Antibacterial	Circulatory
Antidiarrhea	Cleansing
Antiepileptic	Digestive
Anticonvulsant	Disinfectant
Anti-fungal	Diuretic
Anti-inflammatory	Expectorant
Antimicrobial	Hypotensive
Antimucolytic	Laxative
Antiparasitic	Respiratory
Antiseptic	Sedative
Antispasmodic	Stimulant
Anti-viral	Vasodilators

While this list is impressive, it is not to infer that one should use essential oils to treat or cure, but to add to a healthcare regimen, to support health and wellness, remembering to consult medical providers for the treatment of specific conditions or situations.

Essential oils support the body in healing itself.

The purpose for including this information here is so that we are reminded to give our essential oils the respect that they deserve. It is important that we are aware of and always remember the power that just a drop of an essential oil can have. When we do, we will be conservative, yet consistent in use of our essential oils, valuing each small drop, what it contains, and also considering any suggested cautions.

Since it is research that has given us the information that we have about the components in essential oils and their uses or actions, it is important to understand one of the difficulties inherent in this type of study. In doing research and studying essential oils it has been difficult to isolate one component of an essential oil to study because essential oils come in combinations in nature. The benefits achieved are often realized as a result of the synergy we find in the way that nature combines the various constituents of each plant and therefore each essential oil (Schnaubelt, 2012). This is a bit like trying to figure out which ingredient in a recipe makes it taste good when it is the combination of them all!

V: Vaporizer or Humidifier, Hot Water Vapor

This terminology can be a bit confusing, can't it! The devices that disperse essential oils into the air are called by a variety of names: diffusers, nebulizers, humidifiers, and vaporizers. The devices that do best are those that use water with a few drops of essential oil and that break down the particles into the smallest size without using heat, which can reduce the therapeutic benefits of the essential oils. The best devices are those that use ultrasonic vibration. These devices disburse the oil and water into the finest mist, which helps the oil remain in the air for extended lengths of time. It is good to read the description of what the manufacturers state that the device does, and select those that follow these guidelines.

Hot water vapor, on the other hand, is where you put 1 – 3 drops of an essential oil into hot water and inhale, often leaning over a sink or basin with a towel over your head to keep the vapor from escaping. The heat could reduce some of the benefits of the oil, but could help open the nasal passageways and is often used for that reason.

W: Wellness and Essential Oil Use

The use of aromatherapy and essential oils in a holistic program of wellness is often a component of complementary and alternative health practices. It is becoming more commonplace within Western medical understanding as well. The thing to keep in mind is that it is important to also build a solid foundation of health. If using oils is the only thing that a person does to improve their health, they may have some good results, but with a good overall wellness plan, imagine how much they could really accomplish for their health!

The foundation of health is based upon a combination of healthy habits. Consider the interplay between our nutrition, relationships, spirituality, exercise or physical movement, career and other daily pursuits, on our overall wellness and enjoyment of life. If one area of life is out of alignment, it can be much more difficult to improve a specific health concern, or prevent illness. Sometimes, huge gains can be obtained by simply making changes in career or relationships, even without doing anything else!

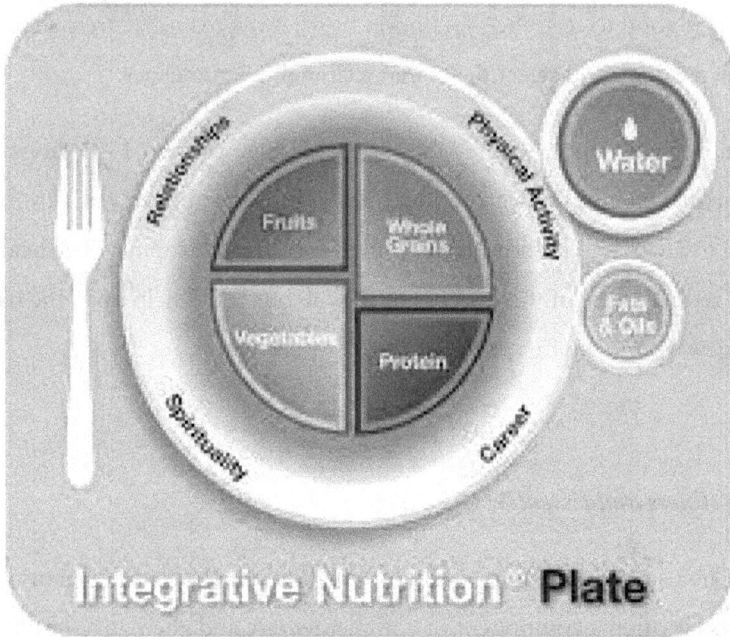

© 2011 Integrative Nutrition (used under license)*

Integrative Nutrition ® Health Coaches are trained to support individuals who seek health and wellness, healing and healthy balance in their lives. Having someone walk beside you and guide you, in finding your best path, can be truly an exciting journey. It is good to have a partner to hold you accountable for the changes and goals you make and a coach can do that for you. Other Certified Health Coaches can also give good support and guidance.

A good place to begin is to take an honest look at where you are. Are there things that you commonly eat that are processed, contain sugars or other chemicals, or that have a long list of ingredients that you can't pronounce? If so, try to replace them with something similar that you cook yourself instead, or a healthier version of that food if it is something that you enjoy. If you hate your job, or are not exercising, or there is stress in some part of your life, consider how you can change that as well.

Consider the categories from the Integrative Nutrition Circle of Life™:

- Career
- Education
- Health
- Physical Activity
- Home Cooking
- Home Environment
- Relationships
- Social Life
- Joy
- Spirituality
- Creativity
- Finances

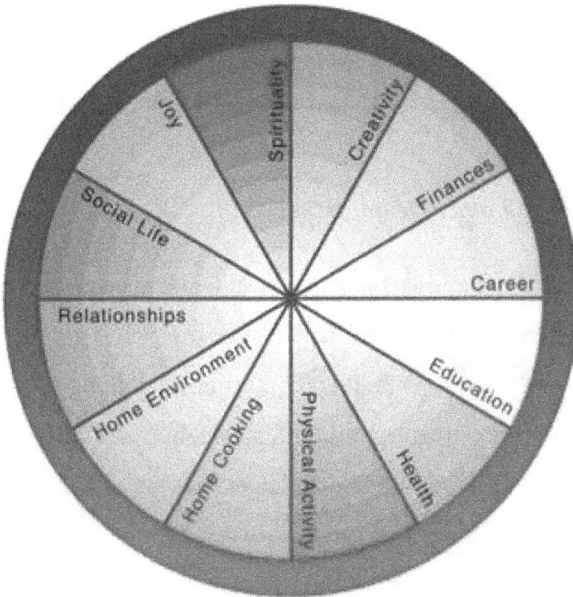

© 2011 Integrative Nutrition Inc.

© 2011 Integrative Nutrition (used   under license)*

If you rate your current status on a scale of 1 – 10, with regard to each of these categories and how well you feel that you are doing in each of them, you can begin to see where you will want to devote some effort to create a balance. Again, having a coach to guide you in how to achieve a comfortable and healthy balance is often needed as it can be difficult to be objective or see our "blind spots" or patterns that could keep us from being successful on our own.

Becoming healthy is a wonderful goal. Consider that it is best to take small steps that can lead to lasting changes rather than make goals with huge changes that you may be unable to maintain for the long haul. Spirituality and meditation or yoga practices can be important and help you tune in and gain insight into what is best for you at any given moment.

*The Circle of Life Design™, Integrative Nutrition ®, and the Integrative Nutrition™ Plate Design are trademarks that are owned by Integrative Nutrition Inc. (used under license).

X: Xerostomia and other Dental Issues

Having spent many years working as a dental hygienist, a common complaint I often heard from our patients was that they had dry mouth, a condition called "xerostomia." It is most common among those who take prescribed medications regularly. Drinking alcohol, not drinking adequate water, or consuming foods containing large amounts of sodium and other chemicals, are other things that can lead to dry mouth. Some believe that the laurel sulfate in traditional toothpastes can also contribute to this condition.

Not only is dry mouth uncomfortable, and can even be embarrassing when speaking to others, it is often accompanied by "halitosis" (bad breath) and can lead to an increase in cavities and gum disease and even periodontal disease. The big issue with periodontal disease (advanced gum disease) is that research has found it to be strongly correlated to heart disease.

Short of stopping taking medications, (not advised without your doctor's approval) there are solutions that have been found to be helpful in supporting oral health and reducing dry mouth and other associated dental and oral problems.

One of the best options I have found is switching to a natural toothpaste specifically formulated with essential oils. Look for one that is free of such chemicals as laurel sulfate and fluoride, and which contains the protective blend as well as hydroxyapatite to strengthen teeth from decay. The protective blend contains essential oils that support healing of the tissues and is soothing as well.

Another helpful solution is oil pulling, which was discussed previously. Oil pulling not only helps remove oral toxins and bacteria, it helps to brighten teeth by removing plaque and stains. Adding a protective blend of essential oils to coconut oil, for example, offers additional benefits when used for this purpose.

The best solution ultimately gets to the root causes of the dry mouth. For this reason, wherever possible, seeking to improve one's overall health to the degree possible is preferred. Often, as people begin to change their diet and add other healthy habits into their lifestyle, they may find that their dry mouth, along with many health issues, will begin to resolve. As health conditions improve, they may even find that their doctors will recommend a reduction in some of their medications or even reducing the dosages, helping even more!

Y: *Youthfulness and Vitality*

When we think of youthfulness, we usually think about energy, health and vibrancy of body and mind. Aging is a natural process, but why give up and give in to all of the ailments and associated difficulties when there are options available to help maintain our health and vitality to the greatest degree possible?

Our doctors help us with broken bones and treating disease symptoms, but our healthy lifestyle choices can make a difference and support our own bodies in doing what they naturally want to do which is find health. Participating in a wellness program that addresses diet, exercise, stress management and sleep, and that helps reduce our toxic load is foundational.

An excellent component in supporting health and increasing vitality is adding supplements that address cellular health, energy and vitality. While it is always preferable to get our nutrients from our food, with the depletion of nutrients in our soil, difficulties in finding organic and nutrient rich options, and reduced or missing digestive enzymes, supplementation can be needed. As we age, we can supplement our diet with nutrients we could be missing, trace minerals, digestive enzymes and probiotics.

Those who take high quality supplements have commented that they experience more energy, less pain, less anxiety and stress and that they sleep better. When we feel better and have more energy, we are more likely to consistently make other healthy changes, such as regular exercise, a good night's sleep, and have an overall improved outlook, increased joy and vitality in life!

and Z... Not the end, just the beginning...

Due to the increasing awareness and interest in essential oils by people from all walks of life, demand for more information is spurring on scientific research, which is growing the knowledge base exponentially. Now, it is easier and easier to find good information at our fingertips. Hopefully this guide will be just like opening the door to a new and exciting vista, providing more hope and guidance for greater joy, vibrant life and abundant wellness.

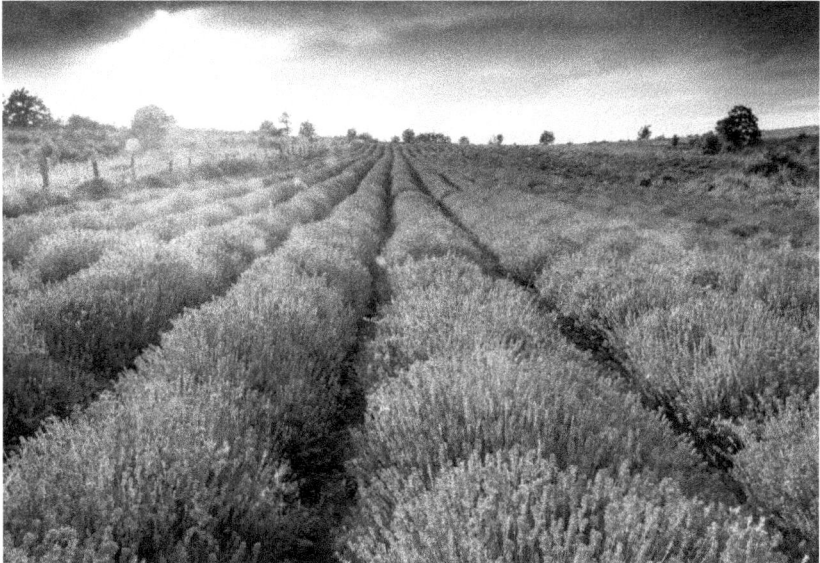

4 REAL PEOPLE: WHAT DO OTHER PEOPLE DO?

Even after going through the 1, 2 3's and the A, B, C's of essential oil use, sometimes we still want to know what other people do. The following is a collection of daily routines by a variety of individuals. Hopefully new users will find a few ideas that you can implement for your own daily use of essential oils.

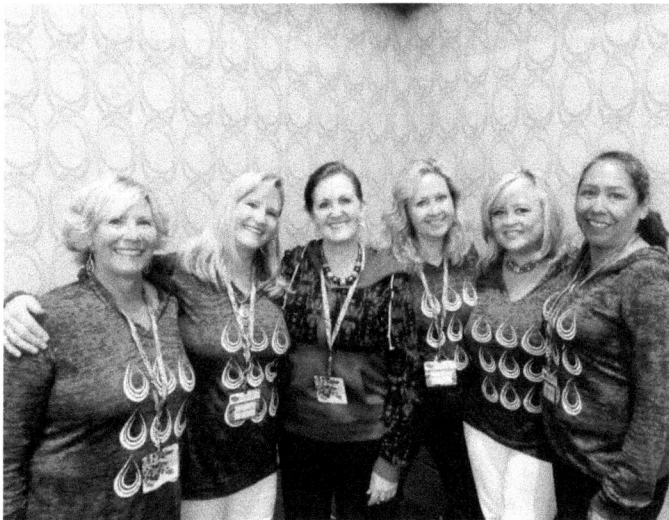

1) An expert on essential oil chemistry and use shared their daily preferences suggesting that we:

- Apply Peppermint and Frankincense to the soles of the feet in the morning to help you wake up, feel energized and ready for the day.

- Diffuse oils such as orange to help invigorate, lighten your mood and protect your home from potential pathogens.
- Apply lavender or other calming or grounding oils to the back of your neck and temples midday to relieve stress. This can be repeated throughout the day as needed.
- Use Peppermint and Lemon in drinking water during the day o help cleanse and detoxifying your body.
- Apply Lavender to bottom of your feet at night or spray on bed linens for relaxation and restful sleep.

2) A teacher suggested:

- *Early morning:* Diffuses a protective blend (3 drops in diffuser) while getting ready and on bottoms of feet before putting on shoes.

  High quality supplements with breakfast.

- *Breakfast:* Green Smoothie with 1 drop wild orange or ginger in it.

  OR hot chocolate with 1 drop peppermint in it.

  OR oatmeal with 1 drop cinnamon.

  1 drop lemon in water several times during the day.

- *At school:* During lectures or testing, 3 drops of peppermint in diffuser. Alternate with a protective blend in the diffuser. If children are agitated, or in preschool for naptime, diffuse lavender for calming.

- *Lunch Time:* 1 drop of lemon on hands to purify.

- *Dinner Time:* Diffuse wild orange for antiviral purposes, or a protective blend if it is flu season. At bedtime, diffuse lavender. A few drops of lavender in a spray bottle with distilled water is good for a linen spray.

3) A nurse practitioner shared:

- I start my day with lemon and a metabolic blend.

- I use a protective blend a lot this time of year. I have it in a spray, and use on hands when I'm out in stores or after each patient I see, etc.

- I diffuse a protective or respiratory blend in the office and at home, keeping the bacteria and viruses of the season away.

- If there are any respiratory ailments rearing, I use a respiratory blend.

- At night I put lavender in my bath... and in my bedroom diffuser in order to create sleep. That's my daily use.

Other people offer their daily routines for using essential oils:

4) I diffuse all day long!

I use:

- A grounding blend on my inner and outer ankles (to regulate my cycle)
- Hand soap (made with a protective blend and cinnamon)
- I use oils on my 8 and 11 year old every night
- 5 drops of lemon in the wash
- Lavender on dryer balls
- Linen spray (for sleep)
- 1 drop protective blend under tongue (have had a tickle in my throat)

I use oils for everything!!!!

5) I love, love, love a grounding blend to start and end the day...

- a female blend for in between....
- clary sage diffused at night to quiet the mind-
- a soothing blend and lemongrass and cypress and white fir for aches and pains...
- then compliment with others as the need arises.

6) I use a grounding blend in the morning on the back of my neck.

- I drink Lemon in my water through out the day.
- I diffuse various oils every day.
- I use wild orange, lavender or the protective blend (one drop) with an unscented hand lotion.
- I use lemon, lavender or a protective blend in the laundry.

- I use lemongrass for joint pain, soothing blend for muscle pain, protective blend with my toothpaste, Frankincense for healing.
- I have various roller ball blends that are used for sleeping, moods, respiratory/cough, restless leg, headaches... digestive blend for GI issues...supplements every day...the list is endless!!!

7) I drink lemon in my water when I wake up

- one drop of Frankincense under my tongue,
- a protective blend in hand soap & for hand sanitizer,
- citrus oils in hand lotion,
- diffuse all day wild orange & cinnamon,
- diffuse lavender at night

8) We are starting off slow.

- We pick one thing & do that for a couple days / week. Or tackle one issue at a time.
- We started with a "flu bomb" for adults (in shot glass of water, gargle, swallow).
- Also put a protective blend on kids feet at night & AM to help them not get sick.
- I just now got all the paraphernalia (rollerball, spray bottles) & am slowly making things.

- And we diffuse when I can remember.

9) We start with a grounding oils and Cassia on bottom of feet at night.

- If I'm not feeling 100% or feel cold coming in ... I use a respiratory blend on my chest and a protective blend behind my ears. Swear by it!!

- Invigorating oils on feet in am.

- We use lemon oil in my homemade body scrub

- If stomach is bothering me I use a digestive blend.

- I take one a protective blend every morning and switch off and on with supplements.

- Vetiver to sleep.

10) My hubby loves this:

- I use (one of the therapeutic layering techniques discussed previously.) And a lot of other protocols in the booklet besides those two. In fact, hubby now requests me to do this more frequently.

11) I agree that it is good to start slow with a few oils and add more.

- Lemon in water is a must for beginners.

- I use the three oils for the allergy bomb (lavender, lemon and peppermint), supplements daily, a protective blend and/or arborvitae on feet if getting sick and vetiver some nights for sleep.

- Sandalwood, cedarwood and patchouli are my choices for diffusing at night. Have fun experimenting!

- Every body is a little different.

12) Overview of our family's use of essential oils:

Myself:

- First thing in the morning, supplements, protective blend, probiotics, 2 drops frankincense under the tongue for depression. Grounding blend and calming blend on wrists. Joyful blend on the back of my neck.
- Diffuse at work either protective blend if someone is sick or joyful blend.
- Lemon in my water all day long.
- Reapply as needed. In the evening 2 drops Frankincense under tongue, supplements, diffuse something all evening and all night.
- Before bed, Clary Sage and Ylang Ylang over abdomen, cilantro and cedarwood on feet.

Whew! And that's if I'm not sick!

Husband: (Back discomfort)

- Daily supplements, protective blend, probiotic,

- For back discomfort: we layer oils on his back. We change it up quite often but right now it's Marjoram, Lemongrass and Frankincense and Wintergreen.

Children:

- 4 year old- protective blend, grounding blend, calming blend, on the back of neck am and pm, Lavender and roman chamomile on feet in the evening.
- 2 year old – protective blend on feet am and pm, lavender and roman chamomile on feet in the evening.
- 4 month old – protective blend on feet am and pm, white fir on gums for teething, lavender and roman chamomile on jawline, lavender on feet in the evening.

13) What we do:

- Supplements daily, diffuse protective blend through day/nite, oils for tension (peppermint, frankincense, and a blend) in my purse as needed through day.
- One child gets oils for supporting respiratory system everyday along with supplements and protective blend.
- Also lavender, lemon and peppermint combined.
- Another child gets Children's Chewables and Omega oil.
- All kids get oils on feet at night and diffusing...usually a protective blend.

14) Our routine:

- Supplements twice daily,
- Frankincense on my tumor and on my arms for muscle pain, along with white fir,
- Anti-aging oils on my face in the mornings
- Cedarwood for sleeping every night.
- Plus many other different oils depending on what is happening in my body.

15) I start with:

- Lemon or orange in my water daily.
- Lavender on my bed, and on my face (diluted) w/ coconut oil.
- Geranium in my face wash, protective blend & peppermint for mouthwash.
- Frankincense on my dog's paws (keeps him calm), I could go on for days!

16) I start with:

- I take a protective blend in capsule each day
- Lemongrass/cypress blend as needed for leg cramps.
- Diffuse whatever sounds good at the time
- I don't overdo any of it, I just take it a day at a time.

17) I use:

- Frankincense under tongue am and pm.

- I also use ylang ylang over my heart twice a day, it keeps my palpitations under control.

- I just use what I am feeling led to otherwise. Here lately it has been the woods...arborvitea, cedarwood, cypress, frankincense...I use them all.

- A grounding blend am and pm on my feet.

18) Well, I'm not your ordinary oiler.

- I have both mental and physical problems and seek support for these.

- Here is how I start the day: lemon in my water to start.

- Next my supplements and herbs for energy.

- Then oils for detoxifying and Frankincense under my tongue.

- Throughout the day I repeat my lemon water adding oils for my metabolism.

- I Take detoxifying oils and Frankincense before each meal.

- I use soothing blend on my extremities and temples.

- Grounding blend and calming blend at night to help me sleep, although I use the calming blend on the base of my neck, wrists and over the heart throughout the day.

- Wild orange and peppermint to wake me up during the day, too.
- Digestive oils as needed.
- I keep my oils close to me!! I have sample bottles in my purse whenever I go out.

19) In AM I start with:

- Supplements, protective blend, 15 drops lemon in capsule and 4 drops frankincense under tongue, grounding blend or lavender on back of neck and forehead.
- Afternoon, vetiver over heart.
- Before bed oils for cellular support, protective blend, grounding blend, calming blend & lavender on bottom of big toes, black pepper on arches of feet, lower back & back of neck.
- Then I diffuse either wild orange, or grounding blend.

Hope this helps!

20) I use:

- Supplements everyday, vetiver and calming blend for sleep, cedarwood in bath.
- White fir for muscle aches.

- Purifying blend and lemon for laundry and cleaning.
- I wear frankincense on a necklace because it makes me happy.
- Lemon in my water.
- Grounding blend on my neck while at work.
- Soothing blend on my lower back and hip.
- Frankincense on my arthritic finger.
- Melaleuca for cleaning and hand sanitizer and owies.
- Protective blend mixed with Dr. Bronners soap in the bathrooms.
- Also peppermint mixed with Dr. Bronners soap.

21) I apply:

- Grounding blend, vetiver, cedarwood, and Frankincense on my son's feet in the morning, making sure I get them all on the bottom of the big toe to help with ADD and depression.
- My 5 year old has allergies and I am following a protocol to hopefully help him get rid of his allergies.... Lemon, Lavender, Peppermint in a roller bottle diluted for his age. Apply to bottoms of feet every am and pm.
- I also apply Melaleuca and lavender layered over his sinuses, and patchouli on the dip at the front of the neck in center of collarbone then I tap 10 times on his thymus (above sternum). I am trying to do this for a year to support in eradicating his allergies.

- I also alternate between lavender and respiratory oils in his diffuser at night.

- I apply Frankincense and grounding blend to the spine or bottom of feet on my 17 year old before sports games and apply what is needed for soreness after or to treat sprains and stuff.

- All of us take supplements. My older kids and hubby take half dose.

- I take the full dosage of supplements, and am using anti-aging oils, oils for cellular support and birch/frankincense roller bottle on hubby for back aches.

- I use soothing blend on any of us if needed.

- Little ones take chewable supplements and omega oil. .

- I use protective blend if getting sick or am sick. I have a roller bottle with respiratory oils and eucalyptus for my 2 year old, one with protective oils, and one with melissa. I use them on her every morning and sometimes at night.

- I use skin care products containing essential oils. The kids use some for teens with acne.

- We use probiotics on and off.

- I use shampoo and conditioner containing essential oils.

- I use a hand wash and cleaner concentrate with protective oils to clean with.

- Diffuse a calming blend in baby's room at night.

- I use different oils every night in diffuser depending on need or mood.

- I use a grounding blend and frankincense everyday.

- I use the allergy bomb (lemon, lavender and peppermint) when needed.

- Digestive blend when needed.

- I use the morphine bomb mix when needed.

- The list goes on. But there are tons you can use them for.

I am an essential oil junkie and proud of it.

Please recognize that some of our "real life essential oil users" mention oils in conjunction with specific health conditions. The oils don't cure these conditions, but they could support the body in healing or soothing itself, along with any treatment they receive from their healthcare professionals.

Now it's YOUR turn! Start your own daily routine and soon you will be your own expert! Remember that it is a process, with some immediate benefits and some that come over time. At the same time, it is such a wonderful world that is opening up to you!

Happy Journey!

APPENDICES

5 APPENDIX A: A, B, C GUIDE TO BASIC ESSENTIAL OILS

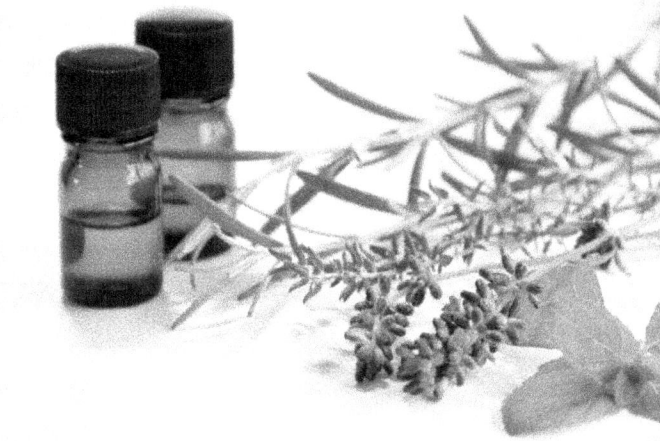

This section includes a list of commonly used, though not exhaustive, essential oils that are good to have on hand.

Key:

T – Topical use

A – Aromatic use

I – Internal use

* - dilute with carrier oil such as coconut oil (1:1) for children and those with sensitive skin

** dilute heavily (1:4 minimally) with carrier oil for topical application

P – photosensitive – wait 12 – 24 hours to go out in sun

Arborvitae: (T, A) The tree from which this oil is extracted is known as the "tree of life," is large, majestic and long living, full of therapeutic properties. Good as a natural insect repellant as it has wood preservative properties, supports against fungal infections, promotes healthy cell function, stimulates and supports a healthy immune system, and protects against environmental and seasonal threats. (Skin, Emotions, Immune System)

Basil: (T, A, I) (Dilute for children and pregnant women)

Basil is a calming oil, that has been found effective in supporting the body with clear breathing, with decreasing the discomfort associated with earaches especially after swimming (with melaleuca), reduces discomfort associated with abdominal cramps, tendinitis, torn muscles, torn ligaments, and symptoms of vertigo. Also good for mental exhaustion. Use sparingly. (Supports Heart, Muscle and Bone Systems)

Bergamot: (T^P, A, I) Promotes emotional balance by restoring confidence and self assurance, and uplifting mood. Aids in reduction of negative thinking, and supports in reducing anxiety and stress. For emotional support, additional benefit can be obtained when combining with lime and sandalwood. Some have found it to aid in appetite regulation. It has also been found to stimulate circulation, support with treatment of psoriasis, acne, cold sores, or abscesses, reduce agitation, and insomnia. (Supports Skin, Emotional Balance and Digestive Systems)

Birch: (T, A) Aids in reducing discomfort associated with cartilage injury, whiplash, muscle aches, as well as supporting the body with muscle development and muscle tone. Emotionally, it supports grounding and calming, can be uplifting and support resilience in the face of life's difficulties. (Muscles and Bones)

Black Pepper: (T*, A*, I) Flavorful in cooking. Often used for smoking cessation support, supports circulatory system, improves digestion, eases aching muscle discomfort, supports alertness and stamina. Good brain support for overcoming negative thinking, encouraging recovery from addiction and healthier new patterns. (Supports Emotions, Digestive, Circulatory and Nervous Systems)

Cardamon: (A, T, I) History as a cooking spice, it is beneficial to the digestive and respiratory systems. Calming for stomach upset, promotes respiratory health and clear breathing. (Supports Digestive, Respiratory Systems)

Cassia: (A, T*, I) Closely related to cinnamon, this oil has a warm fragrance and a lot of historical use. Promotes healthy digestive function, and supports a healthy immune system.(Digestive System, Immune System)

Cedarwood: (T*, A) Promotes healthy skin, is calming, reduces tension, supports healthy immune functioning, supports sleep, and healthy respiratory function. (Supports Skin, Nervous and Respiratory Systems)

Cilantro: (T, A, I) Obtained from the leaves of the coriander plant, it is commonly used in cooking. It supports healthy digestion, and gives food a wonderful flavor. Helps body in reducing anxiety. (Supports Emotional Balance)

Cinnamon: (T**, A*, I) Mostly known for flavor in cooking, it also has many therapeutic benefits. It supports the immune system, circulation, and promotes decrease in discomfort of aches and pains. (Supports immune system).

Clary Sage: (T, A, I) Known best for support of female issues including reducing discomfort associated with menstrual cycles, supports and balances the mood, and hormones. (Supports Hormonal System)

Clove: (T**, A*, I) Used for promoting the reduction of topical pain, especially mouth and tooth pain. Also used topically to decrease discomfort of sprains, strains. Supports respiratory health, digestive health and function, and cardiovascular health. Not only a flavorful spice, it is beneficial for healthy digestive function especially when taken with meals (Supports Cardiovascular, Digestive, Respiratory and Immune Systems).

Coriander: (T, A, I) Support for indigestion, and healthy insulin response, soothes joint and muscle discomfort, supports healthy muscle development, and muscle tone. (Supports Digestive, Muscle and Hormonal Systems)

Cypress: (T, A) Soothing to discomfort with bones, joints and muscles. Supports circulation, and blood flow. Used for greasy, oily hair, and skin revitalizing. (Supports Heart, Muscle & Bone Systems)

Eucalyptus: (T*, A) Used topically to reduce discomfort of sore, tired muscles, or for respiratory health and clear breathing. (Supports Respiratory, Skin Health).

Fennel: (T*, A, I) Used to support healthy digestion, relieving indigestion and common digestive issues. Supports lactation, eases monthly menstrual cycles, and calms minor skin irritation. Promotes lymphatic health. (Supports Digestive and Hormonal Systems)

Frankincense: (T, A, I) Often referred to as the "King" of oils, this one has been around for centuries. It can be added to other oils to enhance their effects. Accelerates skin recovery and healing, including scars and stretch marks. Promotes focus and clarity of mind, reduces irritation, impatience, and restlessness. Supports healthy immune system and function, respiratory and cellular health. (Supports Emotional Balance, Nervous and Immune Systems, Respiratory System, Skin Health)

Geranium: (T, A, I) Hormone balancing, calming nerves and reducing anxiety. Promotes skin and wound health and healing. Good for liver health. (Supports Emotional Balance, Skin Health) .

Ginger: (T*, A, I) Aids overall digestive health including support with nausea, diarrhea, gas/flatulence, morning sickness, vomiting, indigestion, libido (low), scurvy, vertigo, and poor circulation. (Supports Digestive, Circulatory and Nervous Systems)

Grapefruit: (TP, A, I) Used for overcoming addictions, appetite suppression, cellulite, eating disorders, obesity, water retention and stress. Helps decrease mental and physical fatigue. Promotes body cleansing and detoxifying. (Supports Cardiovascular and Digestive/Metabolic System)

Helichrysum: (T, A, I) A precious and highly sought after essential oil, it supports the body in healing of wounds, cuts, scars, irritated skin, and stretch marks when applied topically, helping skin recover quickly. Supports improved localized blood flow, also contributing to its benefit in healing of tissues. (Supports Cardiovascular, Muscles and Bones Systems)

Jasmine: (T, A, I) Beneficial for hoarse voice, Pink eye, sensitive skin, emotional balance. (Supports Emotional Balance, Hormonal Systems)

Juniper Berry: (T, A, I*) Beneficial in many ways, including promoting greater health with problematic skin issues such as dermatitis/eczema. Promotes healthy kidneys and urinary tract. Bolsters the immune system in the healing of colds and flu. Supportive in relieving or reducing tension and stress, and minimizing experience of tinnitus. (Supports Digestive, Respiratory and Nervous Systems, Emotional Balance, Skin Health).

Lavender: (T, A, I) Used primarily for its relaxing and calming properties and wonderful aroma. Used topically to promote speedy healing of skin and to decrease the discomfort of burns, sunburn (with Frankincense), can be soothing to occasional skin irritations from such things as bumps, bruises, insect bites or bee stings. Diffuse or use aromatically for agitation, anxiety, restlessness, agitation and insomnia support. Lavender helps to relax and calm any time another issue is creating distress. (Supports Emotional Balance, Skin, Nervous and Cardiovascular Systems)

Lemon: (Tᴾ, A, I) Primarily known for cleaning, cleansing, purifying properties. Used topically to support healing and to disinfect hands. Use aromatically for healthy immune support. Cleanses the air, reducing stress and fatigue and promoting relaxation. Lemon detoxifies and stimulates the liver. Great for non-toxic household cleaning. (Supports Digestive, Immune and Respiratory Systems)

Lemongrass: (T*, A, I) Used in Asian and Caribbean cooking with subtle lemony flavor and aroma. Aids in decreasing discomfort of sore or achy muscles, and for charley horses (also use with peppermint and a lot of water simultaneously). Purifies and tones skin. Supports healthy digestion. For warming apply to feet bottoms. (Supports Digestive, Immune System, Muscles and Bones, Skin Health)

Lime: (T^p, A, I) Use to promote healing of bacterial infections, fever, and to support healthy immune function. Good for gum/grease removal, and for skin revitalizing. As with most citrus oils, supports positive mood. Stimulating and refreshing, it promotes emotional balance and well being. (Supports Digestive, Immune, and Respiratory Systems)

Marjoram (Wintersweet): (T*, A, I) Used to soothe tired, stressed muscles, supports reduction of discomfort associated with arthritis, rheumatism, neuralgia, and restless leg. Support for healthy respiratory system, and beneficial to cardiovascular system. Calming to nervous system. (Supports Healthy Heart, Muscles and Bones.)

Melaleuca (Tea Tree): (T, A, I) Known best for cleansing and positive effect on skin. Promotes healing of minor skin irritations such as insect bites, itching, sores, ringworm, psoriasis, eczema, and fungal infections. Promotes healthy immune functioning protecting from environmental and seasonal threats such as bacterial (with oregano), viral, as with colds, cold sores, coughs, sore throat, and flu. Some use to remove slivers (combine with clove to draw them out). (Supports Immune and Respiratory Systems, Muscles and Bones, Skin Health)

Melissa (Lemon Balm): ((T, A, I) A rare and valuable oil, this is strongly calming for emotional issues. Promotes healing of viral infections, cold sores, coughing, bronchitis, asthma, skin irritations including eczema, as well as supporting the body in minimizing discomfort associated with migraine, menstrual cramping, and nausea. Beneficial as an insect repellant. (Supports Emotional Balance, Skin Health)

Myrrh: (T, A, I) Promotes emotional balance and well being. Specifically, supports female hormonal balance associated with amenorrhea. Soothing to skin. Promotes healing of minor skin issues such as athlete's foot, chapped skin, and found beneficial in supporting the healing of hemorrhoids, ringworm, and stretch marks. Some indication that it supports healing of gum disease, and ulcers. (Supports Hormonal, Immune and Nervous Systems, Skin Health)

Oregano: (T**, A, I) Use diluted – **dilute with olive oil or coconut oil** – as a cleansing agent, supporting healing of digestive and respiratory functioning. For internal use, drip into capsules or use topically on bottoms of feet, to promote healing and to provide a good source of antioxidants. Also used to promote healing of fungal infections, and in reducing discomfort of inflammation associated with arthritis, backache, bursitis, carpal tunnel syndrome, rheumatism, and sciatica. (Supports Immune and Respiratory Systems, and Healthy Muscles and Bones)

Patchiouli: (T, A, I) Used to promote emotional grounding and balancing. Used as an insect, mosquito and termite repellant. Supports healing of skin irritations associated with acne, athlete's foot, chapped skin, dermatitis, eczema, mature skin and for hair care. (Supports Skin Health)

Peppermint: (T*, A, I) Used to decrease discomfort of topical pain due to bumps, bruises, headache, for cooling of fever, or for digestive issues, including motion sickness, nausea and vomiting, or indigestion. Improves circulation. Beneficial for fatigue or exhaustion, and a good afternoon pick-me-up, or for increased focus. For a stuffy nose, mix 1 drop with a teaspoon of honey and hold at back of throat in mouth until vapor moves into back of throat. (Supports Digestive, Nervous and Respiratory Systems, Skin, Muscles and Bones)

Roman chamomile: (T*, A, I) Primarily known for its calming and relaxing benefits to skin, mind and body. Decreases discomfort associated with bee stings, insect bites, abscesses, boils, cuts, cystitis, inflamed skin, blisters, sores, sprains, strains, stress or wounds. Promotes detoxification, and supports reduction of symptoms associated with PMS, menopause, and allergies. (Supports Emotional Balance, Nervous System, Skin Health)

Rosemary: (T*, A, I) Beneficial for support in reducing cravings associated with additions (alcohol). Stimulating when experiencing fatigue or exhaustion. Good for greasy/oily hair, or to support recovery from hair loss. Helps reduce discomfort associated with headaches, aching muscles, arthritis, muscle cramping and neuralgia. Supports healthy digestion. (Supports Immune, Respiratory and Nervous Systems)

Sandalwood: (T, A, I) Known for its wonderful aroma, sandalwood enhances the mood. It promotes smooth, healthy skin, reducing appearance of scars and blemishes. It supports healthy emotional balance of ADD/ADHD, absentmindedness, depression, and stress. Supports reduction of discomfort associated with back pain. Supports healing and repair of cartilage. (Supports Emotional Balance, Muscles and Bones, Nervous System, Skin Health)

Thyme: (T**, A, I) Promotes healthy inflammatory and immune system response to promote healing of environmental threats particularly during the winter time. Cleansing and clarifying benefits to skin. Used to support healthy hair growth (due to loss resulting from fragile hair). (Supports Immune System, Muscles and Bones)

Vetiver: (T, A, I) Promotes healthy emotional balance and calming for depression, hyperactivity, absentmindedness, and minor memory loss. Supports healing with immune-enhancing properties for acne, arthritis, cuts, and minor sores. Sometimes used as a termite repellant. (Supports Emotional Balance, Hormonal and Nervous Systems, Skin Health)

White Fir: (T*, A, I) Most often used in soothing and decreasing the discomfort associated with bursitis, cartilage inflammation, frozen shoulder, muscle fatigue, muscle pain, overexercised muscles, and sprains. Promotes healthy respiratory functioning and clear breathing. For emotional use, it is energizing to the body and mind. (Supports Healthy Bone and Muscle, and Respiratory System)

Wild Orange: (T^p, A, I) Beneficial in promoting emotional balance and lifting mood. Energizing to mind and body. Supports immune system in protecting against environmental and seasonal issues. Promotes cleansing and purifying. (Supports Digestive, Immune Systems, Emotional Balance, Skin Health).

Wintergreen: (T*, A) Recognizable aroma and taste have been used in candy and chewing gum. Therapeutic benefits include topical use to soothe or decrease discomfort of achy muscles and joints. Promotes healthy respiratory functioning. (Supports Healthy Muscles and Bones).

Ylang Ylang (T, A, I) Promotes healthy emotional balance for anxiety, depression, exhaustion, fear, and stress, lifting the mood. Beneficial in calming, relaxing and soothing for colic and emotional distress. Promotes hormonal balance associated with low libido and frigidity. (Supports Emotional Balance, Cardiovascular and Hormonal Systems)

*This information contained herein was obtained from a variety of essential oil encyclopedias, and texts (titles found in the reference section), and should **not** be taken as medical advice, nor is it intended to diagnose, treat, cure or prevent disease. Please always consult with your physician.

6 APPENDIX B: A, B, C'S OF SUPPORT FOR BODY SYSTEMS WITH ESSENTIAL OILS

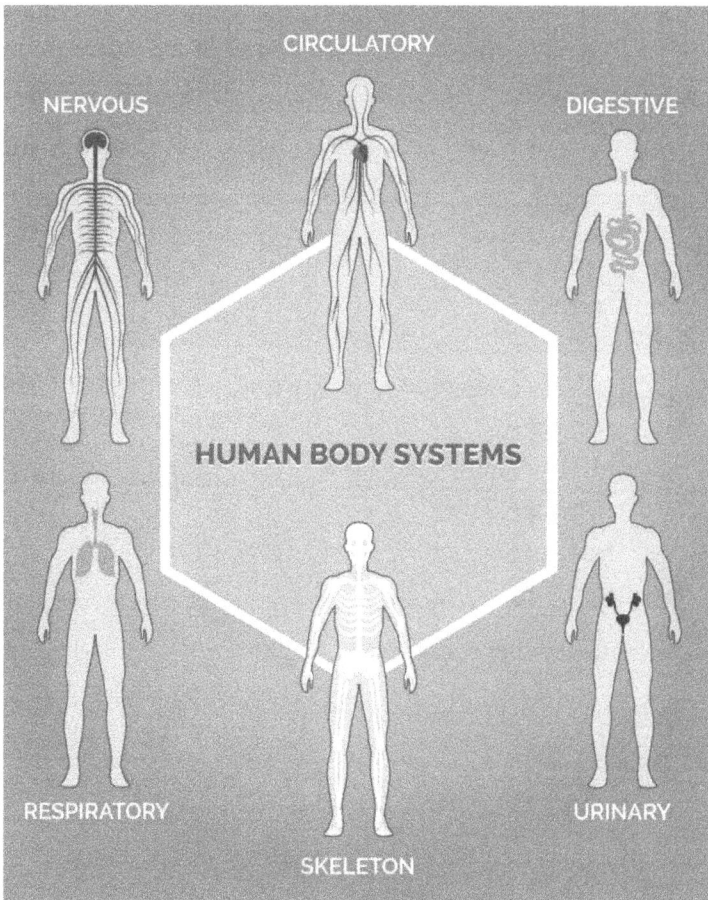

The information contained in this section is a compilation of suggestions for how to support normal body functions and processes through the use of essential oils and essential oil based supplements and products. This information has been compiled from a variety of individuals, encyclopedias, books, articles, and writers, as found in the References section. *For serious health concerns or disease processes, please seek professional medical attention and treatment.

The key when seeking greater health and wellness is that when the body as a whole is functioning optimally, the functioning of all body systems are able to improve and function better. For this reason, in most instances, a foundation of high quality supplements, digestive enzymes and probiotics are recommended. Even eating a highly raw, planted-based diet is most likely lacking in these critical elements as a result of the condition of our soil.

Adrenal support:

Suggested Oils: Clove, Coriander, Cypress, Geranium, Rosemary, Ylang Ylang

Other Options: Basil (renewal), Lavender, High quality supplements for immune support foundation, digestive enzymes and probiotics

Addiction Recovery Support:

Suggested Oils:

- *Cravings:* Clove, Cilantro, Cinnamon, Grapefruit, Peppermint, Grounding Blend, Calming Blend
- *Anxiety:* Grounding Blend, Lavender, Calming Blend, Ylang Ylang
- *Withdrawal:* Lavender, Grapefruit, Marjoram, Sandalwood, Wild Orange, other citrus oils

Other options: High quality supplements for immune support foundation, digestive enzymes and probiotics

Also Consider:

- *Alcohol:* Helichrysum, Rosemary
- *Caffeine:* Basil
- *Drugs:* Grapefruit, Roman Chamomile. (*Marijuana:* Basil)
- *Food:* Grapefruit
- *Pornography:* Frankincense, Helichrysum
- *Sex:* Geranium, Sandalwood
- *Sugar:* Grapefruit
- *Tobacco:* Black Pepper, Clove
- *Workaholic:* Basil, Geranium, Lavender, Marjoram, Wild Orange, Ylang Ylang

Bad Breath:

Suggested Oils: Peppermint, Wintergreen

Bone Health Support:

Suggested Oils:

- Normal Discomfort - Wintergreen

111

- Bone Health Support - Birch (bone healing support), Cypress (circulation support), Helichrysum (support of overall tissue regeneration and repair), Lemongrass (ligament support), Marjoram (tissue rebuilding support), and White Fir (anti-inflammatory support)
- Stress /Tension support - Lavender

Other Options: Clove, Eucalyptus, Frankincense, Ginger, Oregano, Vetiver, High quality supplements for bone support

Breast Feeding Support:

Suggested Oils:

- Increasing milk supply: Clary Sage, Fennel, Geranium (Note: Some report decrease in milk supply with Peppermint, so to be sure, avoid this essential oil or blends containing it)
- Decreasing milk supply: Peppermint
- Sore nipples: Lavender, Helichrysum, Roman Chamomile

Other recommendations: High quality supplements for immune support foundation, digestive enzymes and probiotics

Other Oils Safe to Use During Lactation: Bergamot, Invigorating Blend, Clary Sage, Grapefruit, Geranium, Lavender, Lemon, Melaleuca, Patchouli, Roman Chamomile, Sandalwood, Calming Blend, Wild Orange, Ylang Ylang.

Circulatory System Support:

Suggested Oils:

- *Support for Calming:* Cassia, Clary Sage, Frankincense, Helichrysum, Lavender, Lemon, Marjoram, Ylang Ylang
  Other Options: Clove, Eucalyptus, Wintergreen, High quality supplements for immune support foundation.

- *Support for Stimulating:* Cypress, Geranium, Rosemary
  Other Options: Helichrysum, Lemon, Lime, Peppermint, Rose, Thyme

Cognitive and Brain Support:

Suggested Oils: Frankincense, Lavender, Melissa, Patchouli, Peppermint, Rosemary, Ylang Ylang

Essential oil based products: Massage Blend Technique, High quality supplements for immune support foundation

Other Options: Basil, Cassia, Cinnamon, Clove, Cypress, Helichrysum, Marjoram, Myrrh, Oregano, Sandalwood

Dental Support, Gum and Mouth Health:

Suggested Oils : Clove, Lavender, Lemon, Melaleuca, Myrrh

Essential oil based products: High Quality Toothpaste containing essential oils

Other Options: Eucalyptus, Helichrysum, Frankincense, Peppermint, Rosemary, High quality supplements for immune support foundation

Digestive System Support:

Suggested Oils: Coriander, Dill, Fennel, Ginger, Peppermint

Other Options: Basil, Cinnamon, Eucalyptus, Frankincense, Grapefruit, Lavender, Marjoram, Myrrh, Roman Chamomile, Rosemary, Thyme, Wild Orange,

Also recommended: Digestive Enzymes, Probiotics, High quality supplements for immune support foundation

Emotional Balance Support:

Suggested Oils: Cassia, Clary Sage, Cypress, Frankincense, Geranium, Lavender, Melissa, Marjoram, Patchouli, Sandalwood, Vetiver, Wild Orange, Ylang Ylang

Other Recommendations: Massage Blend technique, High quality supplements for immune support foundation

Other Options: Basil, Grapefruit, Lemon, Rosemary, Thyme

Consumers share the benefits of essential oils for the following normal emotional experiences (Note: Not as related to emotional disorders or treatment, or as a substitute for medical care):

Abundance – Abundance, Tangerine, Ylang Ylang, Lemon, Peppermint

Acceptance – Bergamot

Anger / Irritability –Grapefruit, Patchouli

Cheer / Creativity – Tangerine, Wild Orange, Ylang Ylang, Roman Chamomile, Lime,

Clarity – Clary Sage

Cleansing – Lemongrass, Melaleuca, Thyme, Clary Sage

Communication – Lavender, Lime, Cassia

Connection – Marjoram, Cedarwood, Geranium

Emotional protection – Frankincense

Emotional release – Geranium highly recommended plus Basil, Cassia, Cypress, Melissa, Cilantro, Thyme

Empowerment – Ginger, Clove, Fennel, Helichrysum, Melaleuca

Feminine Energy – Ylang Ylang or Sandalwood, Myrrh, Geranium, Bergamot

Focus – Lemon, Rosemary

Forgiveness –Thyme

Generational Health – White Fir, Birch, Cedarwood

Grief –Geranium,

Grounding/ Centering –Vetiver, Patchouli, Myrrh, Birch

Honesty- Frankincense (Truth)

Hurt / Pain, Surrendering – Helichrysum, Ginger, Wintergreen

Intuition – Ylang Ylang, Tangerine, Wild Orange, Rose, Geranium

Joy- Peppermint

Knowledge / Change – Rosemary, Lemon

Love / Trust – Geranium, Marjoram, Ylang Ylang, Rose

Nurturing- Ylang Ylang, Myrrh (mother/child bond)

Paranoia – Bergamot, Vetiver

Purification –Lemongrass, Thyme, Cilantro

Passion –Cinnamon (sexual)

Protection –Clove, Ginger

Relaxation / Relief – Cypress, Basil, Peppermint

Renewal – Basil

Responsibility- Vetiver, Fennel

Restful Sleep – Juniper Berry, Clary Sage, Black Pepper, Vetiver
Self-Acceptance: Bergamot, Cassia, Melissa
Self Confidence- Frankincense, Frankincense/Peppermint, Vetiver
Self Image –Bergamot
Self Love- Clove (boundaries)
Spirituality / Worship – Roman Chamomile, Frankincense, Melissa, Sandalwood, Myrrh
Support – Birch, White Fir, Cedarwood, Juniper Berry, Wintergreen
Surrender – Wintergreen, Sandalwood, Birch, Eucalyptus, Frankincense
Wellness – Eucalyptus, Helichrysum
Zest/Enthusiasm – Lime, Tangerine, Melissa, Melissa

Focus Support:

Suggested Oils: Clary Sage, Frankincense, Lavender, Vetiver, Ylang Ylang

Additional Recommendations: High quality supplements for immune support foundation

Other Options: Basil, Dill, Marjoram, Patchouli

Immune System Support:

Suggested Oils: Frankincense, Geranium, Lavender, Melaleuca

Essential oil based support: Massage Techniques

Other Options: Clove, Helichrysum, Lemon, Melissa, Oregano

Additional recommendations: Digestive Enzymes, Probiotics, High quality supplements for immune support foundation

Healthy Hair Support:

Suggested Oils: Cedarwood, Lavender, Lemon, Peppermint, Rosemary, Blend for Women

Essential oil based products: Essential Oil Based Shampoo, Conditioner

Other Options: Clary Sage, Cypress, Roman Chamomile, Sandalwood, Thyme, Wintergreen, Ylang Ylang

Also recommended: High quality supplements for immune support foundation

Inflammation and Injury Support:

Inflammation is the body's normal response to a variety of conditions including infection, injury, allergy, and more. The first step is to seek understanding as to the root cause of the problem, seek medical advice, and then use suggested essential oils to support the body's natural processes.

Suggested Oils:

Most mentioned: Frankincense, Helichrysum, Myrrh, Melaleuca

Also mentioned: Basil, Eucalyptus, Ginger, Lavender, Peppermint, Wintergreen

Essential oil based support: Massage Technique

Other Options: Blue Tansy, Cassia, Cilantro, Cinnamon, Citrus Oils, Clary Sage, Clove, Coriander, Fennel, Geranium, Jasmine, Lemon, Lemongrass, Melaleuca, Melissa, Oregano, Patchouli, Roman Chamomile, Rose, Sandalwood, Thyme, Ylang Ylang

Additional recommendations: High quality supplements for immune support foundation

Muscle Health Support:

Suggested Oils: Birch, Eucalyptus, Lavender, Lemon, Marjoram, Myrrh, Peppermint, Rosemary, Wintergreen

Other Options: Frankincense, Ginger

Nerve and Nervous System Support:

Suggested Oils: Cypress, Geranium, Helichrysum, Juniper, Peppermint, Roman Chamomile

Other Options: Basil, Birch, Cassia, Clove, Coriander, Eucalyptus, Frankincense, Grapefruit, Lavender, Lemon, Lemongrass, Marjoram, Oregano, Patchouli, Vetiver, Wintergreen

Additional recommendations: High quality supplements for immune support foundation

Respiratory system:

Suggested Oils: Eucalyptus, Frankincense, Lemon, Peppermint

Other Options: Cinnamon, Clove, Oregano, Sandalwood, Wild Orange

Additional recommendations: Digestive Enzymes, Probiotics, High quality supplements for immune support foundation

Sleep Support and Prophylaxis:

Suggested Oils: Clary Sage, Frankincense, Lavender, Ylang Ylang

Other Options: Marjoram, Roman Chamomile, Rosemary, Wild Orange

Skin Health Support:

Suggested Oils: Geranium, Lavender, Melaleuca

Other Options: Frankincense, Grapefruit, Helichrysum, Lemon, Myrrh, Roman Chamomile

Tension and Stress Management and Support:

Suggested Oils: Frankincense, Lavender, Peppermint, Wintergreen

Other Options: Basil, Clove, Eucalyptus, Ginger, Lemon, Lemongrass, Marjoram, Rosemary

Suggested Protocols:

A drop or two of the selected oil rubbed on the temples, forehead, and/or back of neck. A roll-on with single or blends of selected oils is helpful and convenient. Repeat as often as needed and as schedule permits. A damp compress with a few drops applied to the towel can help the effect last longer. (Keep oils away from the eyes).

Many appreciate the combination of Frankincense, Lavender and Peppermint both applied to temples, back of neck and crown of head as well as diffused and inhaled.

Some find that a personal inhaler is helpful.

Since we all respond differently, rotate or try different oils in your routine.

Weight Management:

Suggested Oils:

Basic: Cinnamon, Ginger, Grapefruit, Lemon, Peppermint

Appetite Suppressant: Dill, Grapefruit, Patchouli

Attitude: Cypress, Oregano, Peppermint, Lavender, Ylang Ylang

Metabolism: Eucalyptus, Grapefruit, Peppermint, Rosemary

Fat Burn: Basil, Lavender, Cypress, Grapefruit

Diuretic: Cypress, Fennel, Lavender, Lemon, Oregano, Rosemary

Additional recommendations: Digestive Enzymes, Probiotics, High quality supplements for immune support foundation

7 APPENDIX C: ESSENTIAL OILS FOR DOGS

Calming Blend. May contain some or all of the following EOs: Tangerine, Orange, Ylang Ylang, Patchouli, and Blue Tansy, lavender, marjoram, Roman chamomile, sandalwood, and/ or vanilla bean	Stress, anxiety, fear, stress associated with pain, separation anxiety
Digestive Blend. May contain some or all of the following EOs: peppermint, ginger, tarragon, fennel, caraway, coriander and anise oils	Digestive issues such as diarrhea, constipation, vomiting, upset stomach, lack of appetite, motion sickness, parasites in GI tract
Eucalyptus	Breathing issues, respiratory ailments (cold, flu), allergies, kennel cough
Frankincense	Wound healing (including suture sites), infections (bacterial, viral, fungal), yeast, scar reduction, calming, skin issues, pain, inflammation, immune support, tumor reduction

Grounding Blend. May include some or all of the following EOs: Spruce, Ho Wood, Frankincense, Blue Tansy, and Blue Chamomile	Calming for dogs that have more intense issues with stress, anxiety or fear
Helichrysum	Stops bleeding, closes wounds (liquid sutures), pain, fungal infection, inflammation, nerve damage, bruises and swelling
Lavender	Skin issues, burns, infections (bacterial, fungal, and viral), wounds, inflammation, calming, disinfects, insect bites, ear infections, allergies
Lemon	Stops bleeding, cleans surfaces, allergies, antibacterial, antiviral, insect repellant, stress, cough, sore throat
Peppermint	Pain, breathing challenges, inflammation, insect repellant, fever, overheating, motion sickness, nausea, indigestion, allergies
Protective Blend. May contain some or all of the following EOs: orange, lemon, clove, cinnamon, eucalyptus, and/ or rosemary	Bacterial infection, yeast or fungal infection, viral infection, immune system support, topical disinfectant (counters or surfaces), neutralizes bee and insect sting toxins

Always make sure that you are using 100% pure therapeutic grade essential oils for your pets for the sake of their health and safety.

8 REFERENCES

Aromatic Science: http://www.aromaticscience.com/

   Research and information on the science behind essential   oils.

Aromatools. (2013). *Modern essentials: A contemporary guide to   the therapeutic*

   use of essential oils (5th ed.). Aromatools: Orem, UT.

Aromaweb. (2015). Your source for aromatherapy and essential oil

   information. AromaWeb, LLC, copyright 1997 – 2015.

Becker, K. (2012). *Forget everything bad you've been told about essential oils for pets.*

   Retrieved from
   http://healthypets.mercola.com/sites/healthypets/archive/2012/05/14/dr
   -shelton-on-pets-essential-oils.aspx

Burfield, T. (2004). *Opinion Document to NAHA: A Brief Safety Guidance on*

   Essential Oils. (NAHA document no longer available. Cited by NAHA,

   2014, Safety Information.)

Emory, J. (2014). *Should you try oil pulling?* WebMD. Retrieved from

http://www.webmd.com/oral-health/features/oil-pulling.

Enlighten Alternative Healing. (2014). *Emotions & Essential Oils: A modern*

resource for healing. Emotional Reference Guide (3rd Ed).

www.enlightenhealing.com/deo/

Essential Oil University (Dr. Robert S. Pappas, founder)

https://www.facebook.com/EssentialOilUniversity

Fife, B. (2015). Oil pulling for a brighter smile and better health.

Retrieved from

http://www.coconutresearchcenter.org/article%20oil%20pulling.htm

Griffin, M. (2005-2015). *Periodontal disease and heart disease: Brushing and*

flossing may actually save your life. Retrieved from

http://www.webmd.com/heart-disease/features/periodontal-disease-heart-health

Hintze, R. & Lawton, S. (2012). *Living healthy and happily ever after:*

Psychological and physical remedies to jump start healing. Living HEA.

Johnson, S. (2014). *Surviving when modern medicine fails: A definitive guide to essential oils that could save your life during a crisis.* Scott A. Johnson Professional Writing   Services, LLC: Createspace.

Lawless, J. (1995) *The Illustrated Encyclopedia of Essential Oils.* Rockport, MA: Element Books, 60-67.

Lis-Balchin, M. (2006). *Aromatherapy Science: A Guide for Healthcare Professionals.* United Kingdom: Pharmaceutical Press, 101. (See: Smoking Cessation).

MacDonald, D. (2012). *Emotional healing with essential oils (Manual I: Introduction).* Enlighten. www.discovertruthwithin.com

Medical News Today. (2014). What is aromatherapy? The theory behind aromatherapy. Retrieved from
http://www.medicalnewstoday.com/articles/10884.php

NAHA (National Association for Holistic Aromatherapy). (2014). *Safety Information.* Retrieved from http://www.naha.org/explore-aromatherapy/safety

News hour. *Oil as mouthwash?* Retrieved from

http://globalnews.ca/video/1251796/oil-as-mouthwash

Pappas, R. (2014). Dr. Pappas on Essential Oil Chemistry. Retrieved from
https://www.youtube.com/watch?v=eb1fia7kBaA
This video is taken from an annual essential oil conference where he
discusses adulteration and the ways in which essential oils can be
altered.

Pappas, R. (Dec. 19, 2014). *Are essential oils better on the skin pure or in dilution?*
Retrieved from https://www.youtube.com/watch?v=T3enekQT1l8

Pappas, R. (Nov. 15, 2014). *The Chemistry of Essential Oils: Intro and a Brief
History of Aromatics.* Retrieved from
https://www.youtube.com/watch?v=gy5yy82bO6I

Pappas, R. (Nov. 15, 2014). *The Chemistry of Essential Oils: Basic Chemistry
Review:* Retrieved from
https://www.youtube.com/watch?v=M7PgWzHadaU

Pappas, R. (Nov. 15, 2014). *The Chemistry of Essential Oils: Hydrocarbons.*
Retrieved from
https://www.youtube.com/watch?v=kVyFt6i3icQ

*Playlist of Dr. Pappas' chemistry videos from college class at Indiana University in C390: The Chemistry of Essential Oils January 10, 2013: Retrieved from

https://www.youtube.com/playlist?list=PLcQ1l_e7C7xuVV60jTJioVxj07d6GtaYH

Patterson, S. (2014). doTerra essential oils for dogs. Website:

www.thedogoiler.com Retrieved from

http://nebula.wsimg.com/6d9c3fac05cb160d2454629401092ef8?AccessKeyId=C62C510C1ABAFCB8AA96&disposition=0&alloworigin=1

Price, S. (1993). *The Aromatherapy Workbook*. Hammersmith, London:

Thorsons.

PubMed Health. (December 30, 2014). *Aromatherapy and essential oils (PDQ)*.

Health Professional Version. Retrieved from

http://www.ncbi.nlm.nih.gov/pubmedhealth/PMH0032645/

Reflexology on the Front Lines of Health Care. (November/December 1998).

Massage Magazine.

Sanchez, L. (2012). *Essential Oils and Chemical Functional Groups*. American

College of Health Sciences. Retrieved from

https://www.youtube.com/watch?v=9jsjBmnvR-Q

Shelton, M. DVM, Video on Essential Oils and Pets:

http://youtu.be/Jj827fDbpB8 Website: http://www.oilyvet.com/

Sole Response Reflexology and Reiki. *Reflexology: Healing with oils on energy points of the feet.* Retrieved from

http://www.soleresponse.com/blog/reflexology-healing-with-oils-on-energy-points-of-the-feet

Schnaubelt, K. (2011). *The healing intelligence of essential oils: The science of advanced aromatherapy.* Healing Arts Press: Rochester, VT.

Tisserand, R. (1995). *Essential Oil Safety.* United Kingdom: Churchill Livingstone.

Tisserand, R. (2007). *Challenges facing essential oil therapy: Proof of safety.* Retreived from

http://roberttisserand.com/articles/ChallengesFacingEssentialOilTherapyProofofSafety.pdf

Tools: www.myoilbusiness.com and www.aromatools.com

For boxes, bottles, cases, flyers, and more.

NOTES:

NOTES:

ABOUT THE AUTHOR

Dr. Smith began her education in nutrition and wellness while obtaining her bachelor's degree. After years as a dental hygienist and educator, she obtained a master's degree in social work from the University of Utah, became licensed as a Clinical Social Worker in Utah and then California. She obtained a doctorate degree in Counseling Psychology from Argosy University / American School of Professional Psychology. She has counseled countless individuals, couples and families in navigating through a variety of relationship and mental health issues.

Always interested in health and wellness, she recognized the connection between physical and emotional health. She recognized the impact of spirituality and even one's career on their overall experience of happiness in life. In order to bridge the gap between body and mind in her education, she sought training from the Institute of Integrative Nutrition™ and became certified as an Integrative Nutrition Health Coach™.

On a personal level, Dr. Smith has been blessed with a wonderful companion and a family including 9 children and 11 grandchildren (and counting!), as well as 2 fur-kids of the feline variety! She enjoys living in Southern California with regular visits to family and friends who live elsewhere.

www.ingramcontent.com/pod-product-compliance
Lightning Source LLC
Chambersburg PA
CBHW050349280326
41933CB00010BA/1396